Turning Mental Health into Social Action

This book offers a refreshing new approach to mental health by showing how 'mental health' behaviours, lived experiences, and our interventions arise from our social worlds and not from our neurophysiology gone wrong. It is part of a trilogy that offers a new way of doing psychology focusing on people's social and societal environments as determining their behaviour, rather than internal and individualistic attributions.

'Mental health' behaviours are carefully analysed as ordinary behaviours that have become exaggerated and chronic because of the bad life situations people are forced to endure, especially as children. This shifts mental health treatments away from the dominance of psychology and psychiatry to show that social action is needed because many of these bad life situations are produced by our modern society itself. By providing new ways for readers to rethink everything they thought they knew about mental health issues and how to change them, Bernard Guerin also explores how by changing our environmental contexts (our local, societal, and discursive worlds), we can improve mental health interventions. This book reframes 'mental health' into a much wider social context to show how societal structures restrict our opportunities and pathways to produce bad life situations, and how we can also learn from those who manage to deal with the very same bad life situations through crime, bullying, exploitation, and dropping out of mainstream society, rather than through the 'mental health' behaviours.

By merging psychology and psychiatry into the social sciences, Guerin seeks to better understand how humans operate in their social, cultural, economic, patriarchal, discursive, and societal worlds, rather than being isolated inside their heads with a 'faulty brain', and this will provide fascinating reading for academics and students in psychology and the social sciences, and for counsellors and therapists.

Bernard Guerin has worked in both Australia and New Zealand researching and teaching to merge psychology with the social sciences. His main research now focuses on contextualizing 'mental health' behaviours, working with Indigenous communities, and exploring social contextual analyses especially for language use and thinking.

Exploring the environmental and social foundations of human behaviour

Series editor

Bernard Guerin

Professor of Psychology, University of South Australia

Can you imagine that everything people do, say, and think is shaped directly by engaging with our many environmental and social contexts? Humans would then really be part of their environment.

For current psychology, however, people only engage with metaphorical 'internal' environments or brain events, and everything we do somehow originates hidden in there. But what if all that we do and think originated out in our worlds, and what we call 'internal' is merely language and conversations that were also shaped by engaging in our external discursive, cultural, and societal environments?

Exploring the Environmental and Social Foundations of Human Behaviour is an exciting new book series about developing the next generation of ways to understand what people do, say, and think. Human behaviour is shaped through directly engaging in our diverse contexts of resources, social relationships, economics, culture, discourses, colonization, patriarchy, society, and the opportunities afforded by our birth contexts. Even language and thinking arise from our external social and discursive contexts, and so the 'internal' and brain metaphors will disappear as psychology becomes merged with the social sciences.

The series is therefore a-disciplinary and presents analyses or contextually engaged research on topics that describe or demonstrate how human behaviour arises from direct engagement with the worlds in which we are embedded.

In this series:

Turning Mental Health into Social Action

Bernard Guerin

Routledge
Taylor & Francis Group

LONDON AND NEW YORK

First published 2021
by Routledge
2 Park Square, Milton Park, Abingdon, Oxon OX14 4RN

and by Routledge
52 Vanderbilt Avenue, New York, NY 10017

Routledge is an imprint of the Taylor & Francis Group, an informa business

© 2021 Bernard Guerin

British Library Cataloguing-in-Publication Data
A catalogue record for this book is available from the British Library

Library of Congress Cataloging-in-Publication Data
A catalog record has been requested for this book

ISBN: 978-0-367-89814-4 (hbk)
ISBN: 978-0-367-89815-1 (pbk)
ISBN: 978-1-003-02128-5 (ebk)

Typeset in Times
by Newgen Publishing UK

Contents

Figures

Tables

Preface

As I hope the reader will discover, this series of books is not about providing a new theory of psychology, and especially not a 'grand theory', even though the contents might suggest that. It is also not providing a new philosophy, except in a broad sense not related to Western philosophy.

The approach argues, in fact, that words do not have 'meaning' nor do they represent, refer to, or express anyhting, and that argues against the whole Western tradition of philosophy. The only thing words do is to change the behaviour of other people *given the right social contexts*. And that is all this huge collection of words is trying to do.

Most of my words that follow are therefore trying to get you, the reader, to observe the world in new ways; be sensitized to see things you did not see before, and then act in new ways on that basis where appropriate. Most of current psychology, I argue, is just looking in the wrong places for answers and explanations. Because they do not find the answers there, they invent even more abstract words and use correlations to support them, so it looks as if we have discovered something.

The first book in this new trilogy goes back to before the 'cognitive revolution' and shows that the whole reasoning for even having a revolution was mistaken. Psychology took a wrong turn by the assumption that humans must 'go beyond the information given'. Instead, I show how all the subsequent ideas of 'processing information' and 'internal constructions and representations' were really about the social uses of language, and all these ideas and theories can be replaced when we 'turn psychology inside out'. Language use is shown to be externally driven by properly observing all social and societal contexts and realizing that thinking is just language use not said out loud. I then show how we can replace our 'psychology' with the diverse life contexts in which we are immersed, and explore how we can contextualize perception, emotion, and thinking in this way so they do not originate 'inside our heads'.

The second book in this new trilogy shows how the other social sciences have already explored our life contexts, and once we are rid of the current abstract explanations in terms of an 'internal' world, we can merge 'psychology' into the social sciences to form a rich analysis of how humans adapt and become attuned to all of our life contexts. In particular, I explore how our behaviours are now hugely shaped by the modern worlds of capitalism, neoliberalism, and bureaucracy, and how the Marxist frameworks are incompatible with current psychology but can be merged in a contextual approach. Several of the very 'individualistic' ideas embedded in current psychology are then shown to arise directly from our complex social, cultural, and societal worlds, and not from 'inside' us. In particular, I turn the 'psychology' of beliefs, the self, the arts, religious behaviours, and many of the 'individual' phenomena of social psychology inside out, to show their external contexts of origin.

The third book in this new trilogy applies social contextual analysis to the important area of 'mental health'. The behaviours observed in 'mental health' issues are treated here as ordinary behaviours that have been shaped in very bad life situations to become exaggerated and trapped because alternative solutions are blocked. To support the many current attempts to stop using the *Diagnostic and Statistical Manual of Mental Disorders* (DSM), I explore all the individual DSM-listed behaviours and show how they can be shaped by living in bad situations with no alternatives, and are not the result of any brain 'disorders'. The types of bad life situations are explored further, and it is shown that many other behaviours are shaped in addition to the 'mental health' behaviours: violence, bullying, escape, alternative lifestyles, self-harm, exploitation of other people, crime, drug taking. It is suggested that all those people involved in any of these outcomes from bad life situations, professionals, and first-hand experiencers, should pool their expertise and integrate how we can *fix the bad life situations rather than try and fix the person*. Based on these conclusions, interventions for fixing bad life situations are explored, including fixing local issues, fixing those bad social situations that interfere with language use and thinking, and how we might begin to tackle those bad situations produced by our current societal contexts and that are leading to new 'mental health' behaviours: capitalism, neoliberalism, bureaucracy, stratifications, colonization, and patriarchy.

Acknowledgements

The books in this series are a culmination of over 45 years of thinking and researching about these issues, taking every approach seriously, and learning from all of psychology and the social sciences (especially sociology, social anthropology, and sociolinguistics). There are too many people to thank (or even remember) from whom I have learned, so I want to really thank again everyone I have acknowledged in my previous books. You know who you are, I hope. All my students from all my courses have also helped shape my writing when I have used them to try out new ideas and analyses—many thanks.

I also want to thank the staff at Routledge for their belief in this trilogy (and the previous one) and their excellent editing and production work.

A note on referencing

First, each book of the series of six is self-contained, and I have aimed to make them readable alone. However, for those brave souls attempting to see the bigger picture, I use cross-referencing of volume number and chapter in this way: V4.7 refers to Chapter 7 of Volume 4 in the series.

Second, I wish to say upfront that this book comes from reading the work of many researchers and authors across all of psychology and all of the social sciences over many years. In my earlier books I have given hundreds of references to the work of others that has shaped my thinking, even when I disagree. However, I know that referencing slows down a lot of readers whom I would like to take something away from these books that might be of use to them. Many of my intended readers also do not have the privilege of being able to track down the references in any case.

For these reasons, I am being a very bad academic in these books and mostly refer to my own summary works. This current book has been intentionally written so that it can be understood without knowing those earlier books, but to academics (real ones, not me) this causes distress because it looks like I am claiming others' ideas when I use a lot of self-referencing. I certainly do not intend this but having thousands of references interrupting the text causes distress to other readers. This time, I am balancing the distress the other way. You can find the references in my earlier books if needed.

Obviously, where I use or rely heavily on someone's work I cite it and academics can look up all the references if they like and find the sources.

Please do not assume that because I make broad claims and then only cite an earlier summary of my own, that I originated all those ideas and claims. I did not. I am bringing all these ideas from many disciplines together so we can get a new picture of humans and what they do, say, and think. I do not want to interrupt the text by hundreds of references, but please do not get the idea that I believe that I originated everything here.

In fact, the entire theme of this and the other books in the series is that everything we do, say, or think originates in our worlds—our social, societal, cultural, discursive, economic, colonized, patriarchal, and stratified worlds. And that includes my writing these books!

1 The hidden histories of clinical and therapeutic psychology

In Volume 4 of this series, I traced part of the history of psychology but focused on academic psychologies, and in Volume 5 I did a little history of how 'social' context has been systematically excluded from our thinking about almost everything for the last few centuries, including within philosophy and psychology. Most of the books about the history of psychology pay scant attention to both therapies and the clinical applications of psychology, and to the role of society in these histories. But therapies have developed through the same time period and are usually added to histories by claiming (wrongly, I argue) that they have developed by *utilizing* what academic psychology has discovered. I believe this is a myth.

And remember from Volume 4 that psychology was 'invented' as a discipline rather than 'discovered'. It was a new way of talking rather than new observations. We will see here that therapy was a little different, because medical and clinical professionals at this time were given clients to observe who had new behaviours or 'symptoms' that they could not explain; but they made lots of observations of these new 'symptoms', which arose from the societal conditions of modernity. The problem was how they went about explaining this via Pathway 1 (V4.1) and the brain.

In this chapter I will put all these histories together and briefly trace where psychotherapies came from, and why they appeared when they did: *what was it about the late 1800s that both academic and therapeutic psychology needed to be invented, and how was this related historically to the 'disappearance' of the 'social'?*

The upshot is that if you believe that humans create their worlds internally, in their brains or in cognitive processing units, then it is plausible that people's problems or dysfunctions would have been consistent throughout human history and there would be a fixed and permanent set of human disorders. If 'depression' is an inherited problem in the brain or in the cognitive 'architecture', then the vicissitudes of life would not have changed 'depression' over the centuries.

If, on the other hand, like this book, you believe that we are shaped by the worlds we are embedded within and engage with (Pathway 2), then human issues and distress will have been changing throughout history as circumstances changed and the idea that there are fixed 'disorders' is dubious. And even if the same topographical behaviours have occurred over centuries for humans in distress (crying, fear, delusions, etc.), this can occur because there are only a limited number of things humans can do anyway when confronted by bad situations they cannot control. *If symptoms look the same this does not mean they have the same origin or function* nor that they should be treated in the same way. We do not treat crying when really happy in the same way as crying when very sad—the situation determines our response.

What we will find in this chapter, drawing upon a number of historians and sociologists, is that our societal worlds changed drastically in the late 1800s and this produced a whole new set of issues for most members of society, and a whole new set of 'symptoms'. The people affected most by this 'new society', mostly those that were oppressed, were sent to be treated by the medical profession, but these doctors could find no explanations or evidence of brain or neural damage. So, what did they do?

In the history of psychology outlined in V4.1, the Gestalt criticisms of academic psychology were followed by an intensive development of 'internal' discourses about this new domain of 'psychology'. Looking for answers in the worlds in which people were immersed was not considered until more recently. You will no doubt remember that the 'internal' approaches (Pathway 1) that took over psychology from about 1940 onwards had three main responses or discourses:

1. Build neurophysiological models and *promise* that they will one day explain the origins of behaviour.
2. Build hypothetical models and theories of what *might* be going on inside the head (still assuming that is where it all happens).
3. Use everyday common talk and *assume* that we all know what these words refer to (drives, feelings, beliefs, thinking, decisions, choice, will, etc.).

Psychotherapies and clinical psychology today usually assume the first of these discourses (1) in the background, whereas psychiatry makes stronger claims about the brain as the future site of understanding 'mental health' issues. Cognitive behaviour therapy has built its discourses upon the various theoretical models proposed by academic psychologists in line with the second response (2), although it is not clear how far these theories have actually directed or guided therapeutic practices.

But most psychotherapies, counselling, and clinical psychology practice over their short history have fallen in line with the third form of discourse (3) when they talk about case studies and treatments. This is understandable since they must use this same everyday language when talking with clients in any case, but it does not guarantee that any of it is correct. And on their borders are all the 'pop psychologies' that *require* the use of everyday terms to satisfy customers.

In line with this history (V4.1), the medical professionals of the early 1800s proceeded to generate 'explanations' using a weird mixture of invented jargon (2) and everyday expressions (3), focusing closely on assumed brain damage (1) even where none could be found. This is still, to this day, the theoretical basis of the *Diagnostic and Statistical Manual of Mental Disorders* (DSM) and modern psychiatry. Each diagnosed problem is said to be a distinct disease of the brain (1) even though they have never found any damage per se. Others, like Freud, Jung, and later cognitive behavioural therapy (CBT), produced elaborate 'internal' explanations and models (2) of what was going wrong (Guerin, 2019). Still others, like Adolph Meyer (1948), and Karen Horney to some extent (1935/1999), produced 'common-sense' explanations that relied on *everyday ways of talking and explaining* why people do what they do (3).

So, the medical reactions to the inexplicable new symptoms followed the 'internal' explanations linked to promises of brain disorders as done in general medicine. This was historically understandable if, as I and others suggest, *it was the bad life situations arising from changing societal relationships that shaped these new 'symptoms'*, because, as medical professionals, they were never trained to look outside the person for their 'explanations'. And academic psychologists were doing exactly the same during this period but their focus was on the sensory systems rather than the brain at this stage (following Wundt), and did not provide any useful theories or discourses to import into clinical practice (although you can find a few clinical discourses of this time trying to use discourses about the sensory organs and 'inputs', suggesting that something is wrong with your sensory apparatus when you have 'mental health' problems).

Just like academic psychology, then, psychotherapies unfortunately did not react to these new clinical problems by looking more widely at the external contexts from which the behaviours (symptoms) arose, and they did not have the methodological skills to do this in any case (Pathway 2).

However, one strong advantage for those working in primarily medical clinical settings, as opposed to academic psychologists, was that they *did* get to observe more about real people at first hand and at the least talk to them, albeit in an office, hospital, or asylum, and only for a short time period. In this practical realm of real live human beings needing help, they did invent a number of *procedures*, through trial and error rather than through academic theories, and many of these procedural events *did* help their clients even if their theorizing about it was not good (this is well summarized in Janet, 1919/1925). They developed 'talking cures', applications of hypnosis, and many other creative techniques. Later in this volume, I will examine the question of why, when the person's environments were shaping their 'problem' behaviours and it was those environments that really needed changing, these impromptu *talking* therapies even worked at all.

Why did psychology appear at the end of the 1800s? Some social and political contexts

Where did psychology come from? Why was there no psychology before the late 1800s? And why did psychiatry arise from medicine at about the same time? Was that a coincidence?

The common answers are as follows:

- The academic study of humans had at last started using some scientific methods, it became 'respectable' and able to enter the realms of the 'scientific disciplines' (V5.1). These scientific methods were then used to derive the clinical applications.
- Descartes convinced everyone that the answers lay inside people's physiology, but the study of human physiology was so backwards that an intermediate 'science' needed to be invented until we could explain everything by physiology (still waiting … in reality, response 3 took its place, see V4.1).
- The mysterious question from philosophy of awareness or consciousness became a new focus for actual study, and the new academic psychology stopped just talking about it (philosophy) and instead started asking real people to report verbally their experiences (the new academic psychology of Wundt, etc.).

All these are based on typical arguments that decontextualize the social and political history, and make it seem like the 'ideas' are driving history. Michel Foucault (1970, 2009) and many others laid to rest these sorts of narrow approaches in history, so we need to look at the societal history that was going on at the time. And ask instead: What changes were going on in Western society in the late 1800s that the study of how people function became useful, and how was this captured and utilized by those societies? Was psychology even necessary in hindsight?

The social/economic/political context of the birth of psychology

Many factors obviously would contribute to something like the invention/discovery of psychology and psychotherapies. I want to highlight a few of these, but the main mix of contexts were (V5.3): (1) that the final establishment of a fully capitalist economy and vast industrialization were leading to new bad life situations for most people; (2) for obtaining most of their life resources, people now had to form social relationships with strangers held together only by contractual obligations and no longer in familial social relationships that had extensive obligations; and (3) that very large groups of strangers were trying to live together and they needed to be controlled as a whole society. *Remember that all these were occurring for the first time in human history.* Here are some contexts to consider:

- The population, especially in Western countries, was increasing rapidly due to changes in resource production and distribution, and the extra resources brought in from colonization. Westerners were now living in groups (cities) larger than anything experienced by humans ever before, and solutions to the new problems of living like this were still being made up as we went along (they still are).
- Capitalism had ushered in a new era of strategizing the resources of life through stranger or contractual social relationships rather than through families, and once again, solutions to the new problems of living like this were still being made up as we went along. People now spent most of their time and got most of their resources through people they did not know and who had no other obligations or responsibilities towards them or their families.
- The above two points led to a life focused on 'working' for strangers for a single outcome (money), which then was used to get all of the resources of life. You could no longer rely on family to provide resources. *Working and productivity now became the measure of how much people were functional or dysfunctional in their lives.*
- Getting things done and controlled in the wider society also became the responsibility of stranger systems rather than familial systems, which led to the rise of bureaucratic and government systems through which we have to work to get things done in our lives (V5.3).
- Capitalism and the obligatory use of money also led to making the 'individual' become the unit of society (V5.3), and so life outcomes became the responsibility of each individual rather than communities or families. People were on their own and responsible for their

own outcomes. This was basic to liberal economics (and still is) and underlies the rejection of anything 'social' in explaining life (V5.1).

- The use of money, the anonymity of stranger social relationships, and the use of society to control people (bureaucracy, law, government, police), all meant that *the impact of social and societal influences became less easy to identify or observe*. In the past, family were directly influencing people and shaping their behaviour, and this was fairly easy to observe and identify when things went wrong within a family. With the plethora of stranger social relationships, even for children at school by this time (public schools were replacing community or church schools), *it became harder to observe what was shaping both your own behaviour and the behaviour of others*.

- Because of the huge increase in populations living together, governing bodies were rapidly trying to invent new systems to control people, with both good and bad intentions (Foucault, 1970; Miller & Rose, 1994; Rose, 1999). This came to include psychiatry and psychology.

The practical origins of 'psychological' therapies and psychiatry

As mentioned earlier, if 'mental health' issues are truly internal to humans and their brains, then there should have been continuity of 'symptoms' over the centuries. Some of these behaviours show topographical continuity, meaning that similar behaviours have always occurred, but this does not mean that they have arisen for the same (brain) reasons. Just because 'melancholy' looks like the current diagnosis of 'depression' does not mean they are functionally the same at all. Crying in the twelfth century looked identical (I imagine) to crying now, but that does not mean they are functionally the same, and the same applies to crying when you are very happy.

Towards the latter part of the 1800s people started having behaviours that, although some 'resembled' common behaviours, the medical professionals assigned to treat them were at a loss to explain how they were arising. That is, people started presenting with behaviours that caused problems in their lives (e.g. made them 'irrational', V5.1), but there were no easy or obvious reasons why these behaviours were happening.

These new problem behaviours in the 1800s included seemingly unprovoked crying and sadness, limbs becoming rigid, lethargy, tics, doing inappropriate social behaviours, fainting, convulsions, disengagement from the world and from social relationships, conversations and talk becoming unintelligible, and overdramatized behaviours. These all occurred already in human lives, but what was new was that the people themselves and those around them could not identify where they were arising from.

Such 'cases' were given to physicians and medical professionals to deal with by those governing authorities who were trying to control the *large stranger populations* now in existence. People with these 'symptoms' could no longer work or be productive (the goals of capitalism and neoliberalism), nor were they functioning within their families so they could be looked after that way, so they were therefore dysfunctional in these new forms of society. They were handed over to the medical profession when nothing else succeeded in making them productive again.

Because of their training, medical professionals looked for brain or neurological issues with these people, but for the largest proportion nothing could be found. As we saw earlier, at this point three discursive strategies clicked in to deal with this puzzle:

• Attribute what you cannot see to originating in brain processes that will be discovered one day.
• Build theoretical (discursive) constructions or abstract theories to act as 'explanations' for what is observed, including invented jargon.
• Use everyday, common-sense terms and words to 'explain' what is going wrong.

Unfortunately, medical training was such that the full observation and description of these people's *contextual worlds*, including cultural, social, patriarchal, and economic contexts, was not done (Pathway 2). Because they automatically assumed that there must be a brain disorder or other form of internal problem, there was no need to look further. Freud and others did look more closely at *familial* social contexts for the causes of these problems (and found little but Greek myths because the important relationships had switched to strangers by then), but they did not grasp the new and large extent of stranger and bureaucratic systems from the changes in societal foundations.

The history of the therapeutic attempts to deal with these symptoms was therefore a juggling act of the three (Pathway 1) discourses above.

As an early example, in 1852, the French physician Bénédict Augustin Morel wrote his two-volume *Traite des Maladies Mentales*, and in the second edition in 1860 he came up with the term (response 2) 'dementia praecox' (*demence precoce*) for clients suffering from 'stupor' (melancholia). In 1857, he published *Traité des Dégénérescences*, which tried to understand 'mental illness' based upon the theory of 'degeneration', which became one of the most influential concepts in psychiatry for the rest of the century (response 1). The brain and nervous system were said to *degenerate*, and this led to all the symptoms that were appearing. The was no evidence for this degeneration then, or now, but this discursive form of 'explanation' was very influential, despite being vacuous.

To repeat myself a little, the topographical behaviours that were seen by Morel and others, such as stupor and inexplicable sadness, were not new, they had always been there. What was new and really needed changing were the bad situations from which these now arose. To summarize:

- No obvious causes arising from the person's world could be found (because their training was not contextual).
- No common physiological causes could be found, including the brain and nervous disorders already known to medicine.
- No problems or issues from the person's immediate family social relationships could be found (Freud had to promote myths).

The discursive strategies used by the medical people therefore were:

- Talk 'as if' it was a brain or neurological problem regardless of having no evidence ("Their brain has begun degenerating").
- Invent new jargon or theoretical terms ("It is an *unconscious* reaction to a probable underlying conflict", "What this client has is caused by a *psychological* problem in their brain now known to be dementia praecox").
- Use common language to talk about what is going on ("They have really just lost it", "They have gone fully insane, that is what is wrong", "They have a mental illness that is causing this", "They are just mad").

In all three cases, note, the given 'cause' is *purely a discursive strategy* on the part of the physician, not based on observations. One collateral consequence of the abstract verbal nature of all this was that *competition* between the various schools of thought around these issues was made up purely of verbal bluff games, since there was no evidence to debate. This competition therefore became more like who can say their theory the loudest or with the most prestige and status, rather than, what observations do you have? Each of these three types of discourses were verbal and arbitrary and so heated disputes arose since there was no form of observation that could decide who was correct. Territories were drawn up and are still present today. Competition and in-fighting in professional groups and science usually means that observations have not been made (V5.1) and that the statements are being treated as having truth or falsity.

And so it was that several *competing* schools of thought arose in the different hospitals and establishments dealing with these patients, who had been admitted because no obvious causes could be found for their out-of-place and dysfunctional behaviours. The Nancy School and the Salpêtrière Hospital, both in France, were the most important and influential. And most of those physicians working elsewhere with similar clients, including a young Sigmund Freud, visited and studied with these establishments and had to play the politics.

Before writing briefly about these schools, it needs to be noted that earlier, Franz Anton Mesmer (1734–1815) had explored the ideas and practice of 'hypnotism', which he was calling 'animal magnetism'. His practices, also called 'mesmerism', involved touching and pressing on certain areas of a patient's body, leading some patients into convulsions or fits, with 'body fluid manipulation'. Mesmer's animal magnetism became so popular that it quickly spread throughout Europe.

What is important here is that Mesmer and others claimed that such mes-merizing also was able to *cure* some patients' 'psychological' and sometimes physical problems, especially those that did not seem to have an observable cause. And so the vogue of treating patients by having them enter a trance became especially popular in France, and attracted physicians such as Jean-Martin Charcot and Hippolyte Bernheim. Once again (V5.1), we must judge the *events* and *observations* of what these people did to clients very differ-ently from what they *said* about what they did and how they *explained* the outcomes. But this applies to all sciences, even physics and chemistry (V5.1).

What we get to at this point is that new observable forms of 'doing things to help clients' who had new symptoms blossomed (Janet, 1919/1925). They were at least observable and not purely discursive, but all the abstract jargon from responses 1–3 was added on afterwards and then fought over.

Hippolyte Bernheim and the Nancy School

When the medical faculty of the hospital in the French city of Nancy took up hypnotism, about 1880, Hippolyte Bernheim was very enthusiastic, and soon became one of the leaders of the investigation. Bernheim is chiefly known for his theory of *suggestibility* in relation to hypnotism, because he moved away from putting clients 'into' hypnosis to instead using *suggestions* (about getting better) in a waking state. In 1886, he borrowed Hack Tuke's term 'psychotherapeutic action', and in 1891 he used the term 'psycho-therapy' in the title of a book as a synonym for his *suggestive therapeutics*.

What we see here is that instead of using tricks of distraction by hyp-nosis, Bernheim worked just by talking to clients and making suggestions about changing their behaviour. This was the real beginning of talking cures and psychotherapies. It was assumed that changes could be made by talking to clients in their normal state and using the therapist's influence and status to make suggestions about how they might change. Unfortunately, there was still no observation or analysis of the bad situations in which the clients were living, and no analysis of what the therapeutic context itself might be doing.

Bernheim had a significant influence on Sigmund Freud, who visited Bernheim in 1889 and witnessed some of his experiments. Freud translated Bernheim's *On Suggestion and Its Applications to Therapy* in 1888, and also wrote: "I was a spectator of Bernheim's astonishing experiments upon his hospital patients, and I received the profoundest impression of the possibility that *there could be powerful mental processes which nevertheless remained hidden from the consciousness of man*" (cited in Jones, 1953, p. 238, my italics). For Freud these 'powerful mental processes' were turned into abstract, internal 'unconscious' processes (response 2), whereas for myself and others, they were really *hidden societal forces producing bad life situations* that were changing and shaping people in new ways.

Jean-Martin Charcot

The other big influence in these developments was Jean-Martin Charcot, a French neurologist and professor of anatomical pathology. He was known for his work on using hypnosis to treat 'hysteria', especially in his work with a 'hysterical' patient, Louise Augustine Gleizes. The Salpêtrière Hospital in Paris rose to fame under his leadership, because the patients were treated through observation for what is believed to be the first time. They were also not locked up and given some freedoms not found elsewhere.

But Charcot was a physiologist, and therefore conducted careful observations trying to prove an underlying physiological basis for the clients' new and strange behaviours (response 1). He started using modern scientific practices like laboratory analyses, photographs, electrostimulation, drawings, casts, and post-mortem histological sections. He had many young physicians study with him that were later highly influential, including Sigmund Freud, Eugen Bleuler, Alfred Binet, Pierre Janet, and Georges Gilles de la Tourette. While he never found any physiological bases for these new 'mental disorders', he did identify many other neurological disorders and his diagnoses are still recognized today by physicians. These include multiple sclerosis, amyotrophic lateral sclerosis (Lou Gehrig's disease), and Parkinson's disease.

The important observation for 'mental disorders' made by Charcot was that under the influence of hypnosis, and sometimes during an induced fit, patients could lose their symptoms and be 'cured' enough to return to their former lives. What was occurring was not really understood, except for layers of discourse using responses 1–3, but there were some practical results.

Pierre Janet

Pierre Janet (1859–1947) studied under Charcot at Salpêtrière. He developed very modern theories about hysteria, dissociation, subconscious, transference, and a developmental model of the mind's organizational levels. While the latter is sometimes said to have sparked controversy between him and Freud over who first came up with these ideas, if you read their works there was no real controversy. Janet's ideas about dissociation phenomena, for example, are still worth reading now.

Janet's main contribution for this brief history is that he moved the discussion of these new types of 'diseases' from the physiological or neurological to a new way of talking—that of 'psychological' problems. In terms of Pathway 1, he moved the discussions firmly from response 1 to response 2. He was basically saying that we do not *need* to know the details of what is happening in the brain for such cases, because they belong in a realm of 'psychology' that is neither spiritual nor brain-based. This was a useful (at the time) discursive invention, which was made not from new observations or evidence, but from a desire to get away from physiological foundations and other jargons of the day. It also linked with the discourses of Wundt and Titchener in academic psychology and their psychophysical parallelism.

Another important contribution by Janet was his practice of writing up case notes on clients. He had literally thousands of these notes and throughout his writings he gives concrete examples of *observations* he has made to support his theories. While his interpretations might be questioned, his use of cases is enlightening to anyone reading his works for the context provided of individual cases.

A final highlight of Janet's (1919/1925) work, at least for me, is his two-volume 1919 book on 'psychological healing' in which he describes every form of therapy available at that time for these 'psychological' problems. These therapies range simply from prescribing 'rest', to all the therapies of suggestions, early psychoanalysis, early forms of 'mindfulness', distractions, moral imperatives, etc. Reading these volumes really gives you the idea that our current therapeutic techniques have not actually changed that much since 1919 except in how we describe and name them. Most of the 'techniques' of modern CBT are contained in these pages but not dressed up in the current scientific language. Our discourses have changed but the basic practical techniques of attempting to change these symptoms have not. This does not mean that they do not work, just that the discourses do not help.

Sigmund Freud

The final person I wish to mention is better known but perhaps not well understood. He played an important part in the changing *methods* of psychotherapeutic practice as well as further development of the *discourses* around psychology and psychotherapies. Freud had either visited or known the works of Bernheim, Charcot, and Janet. He took discourses and practices from them all but went in some different directions.

He started his work with hypnotism and the 'suggestion' practices derived from Charcot and Bernheim, but he documents how they did not always work for him and so he gradually moved more to *sampling the patients' discourses* rather than distracting them through hypnosis or making suggestions for behaviour change (which were probably hit and miss when they left his office). The *point* of doing these differently in turn arose from the increasingly obvious idea from Janet that: *something or some forces are influencing the clients who have these new symptoms, but what these forces are can neither be easily observed nor can they be talked about by either client or therapist.*

Janet was happy to then talk about these as 'psychological' forces impacting on clients, but this is tautological and gives us nothing beyond Janet's excellent descriptions of clients. Freud went further in his discourses but made abstract theoretical proposals (response 2) instead to try and guide his therapeutic practice. He also did further documentation of these 'unknown' forces (he started calling them the 'unconscious'; Pathway 1) shaping what the clients do, by very creatively including 'slips of the tongue', dreams, and other human phenomena to show that these forces are real.

In this way Freud developed his several theories of an 'unconscious' that partially controls what we do even though we are unaware of it. He observed that in many (or sometimes all) cases of the new inexplicable symptoms, there had been some traumatic event that was 'repressed' by the unconscious so that the client was no longer aware of its influence on them and could not talk about this even though the 'unconscious' could. In general, his technique was based on the assumption that making these hidden, unconscious, repressed thoughts or ideas become conscious (said out loud), would lead to a cure of the symptoms.

So, Freud's basic discursive manoeuvre was to give an invented, abstract name to an inferred 'internal' source that shaped the client's inexplicable behaviours. Once again, because of his medical training, sadly he did not explore the possibility that the origins for these inexplicable behaviours and 'forces' were from the new external societal pressures, or that *these newly created bad societal situations were his unconscious forces* (V5.3). I contend that the unobservable 'forces' shaping these strange new behaviours were in the clients' external worlds and not anything inside of them. Freud obviously had an inkling of this (he saw effects of early life traumatic events), but his later explorations of 'culture' and the wider society were not his best, again because he read mythology and the misguided 'anthropology' of his era, rather than sociology. But once this is realized, a lot of what Freud and Janet wrote about, especially when it comes to the clinical observations, can still be useful if understood as the strong but hidden impact of external societal contexts rather than an 'unconscious' (see an example from Jung in Guerin, 2019).

Since Freud

Since Freud there have been many variations on the way he created a new discourse about these mystifying symptoms arising from *hidden forces*. These have mostly either changed the language or the jargon but are still talking about similar things to Freud (Pathway 1), or else they have invented new practices in clinics that seem to change the 'symptoms' in new ways. But the basic change in thinking or talking about these inexplicable symptoms was set in motion by Janet and Freud. Almost everyone since has been content to wallow in the same discourses of 'hidden internal problems leading to unusual or inexplicable symptoms', rather than seeing the external societal contexts as the source of the issues.

A few people tried to move in new directions when dealing with people with 'psychological' problems (Harry Stack Sullivan and Karen Horney, for example), but the main discourse of 'internal problems leading to external symptoms' has remained despite new jargons being invented. A lot of these later writers, including, for example, the discourses of Carl Rogers and Abraham Maslow, were firmly Pathway 1 but response 3—using ordinary language as if it was a correct description and explanation. I will mention just four important additions to my potted history, however.

Governments and the new psychiatry and psychology

As mentioned earlier, at the same time as the fields of psychiatry and psychology were emerging, those governing our modern societies were looking for ways to control the new large and non-kin-based population. All the above points just mentioned, along with the medical prestige, were sufficiently convincing for them to hand over the *legal control* of people showing unusual and possibly dangerous behaviour with no obvious source to the medical professions (which became psychiatry) and this was later shared with psychology. Hand in hand with psychological 'understanding' (response 3), these clients could be governed by leaving them to the medical profession. So, hospitals and asylums became places to 'dump' uncontrollable people even if there seemed to be no medical symptoms.

Kraepelin and the DSM

The medical discourse in the early 1900s, that the new and inexplicable symptoms were a result of (unknown) brain or neurological damage, was continued strongly by Emil Kraepelin and others and led to the DSM approach to 'mental illness' still used in psychiatry and clinical psychology today. This approach mimics biological taxonomy in the following way (also see V5.1), which I summarize in the following way:

> Every one of these new and inexplicable symptoms arises from some problem in the brain or physiology, a disease or disorder that leads to the unusual behaviour. The idea was that, just like animal taxonomy, if we could only group the 'symptoms' into correlated patterns then we might assume that each of these clusters must have a distinct brain disorder at its root. Neurological research can then use these clusters to identify the source of the problems in the brain.

Unfortunately, there are many discursive and philosophical flaws in the above reasoning, but the medical profession was so strong (having been given that power by bureaucrats and governments) that it led to the now infamous 'standard' ways to group the new symptoms, which are only now being overthrown (Guerin, 2017; Johnstone et al., 2018; Kinderman, 2019; Watson, 2019). Again, those governing the large populations of strangers now accumulated in cities were able to use these 'diagnostic tools' to control parts of the population who were not 'fitting in' to modernity.

Each unusual symptom was said to arise from a diagnosable disease, and each will therefore have a standard treatment once it is identified. This fits perfectly with the more recent neoliberal twists in governing our modern societies: identify the problem and bring in the standard solutions that will fix that problem, every problem has a standard cure/solution. And for those *political reasons*, not because they have actually located any of the hypothesized diseases in the brain, the DSM and the *International Classification of Diseases* (ICD) have now become the standards of mental health treatment.

An issue with this approach is that most time and focus in therapy is now spent on identifying the disease diagnosis from the DSM (V4.7). So actual observations of the person and their life situations and finding answers in the bad situations we now face in our modern social, patriarchal, and economic contexts has been reduced even further.

Psychiatry and drug treatments

Another problem of these developments is that the discursive strategies of the medical professions, which assumed that the odd behaviours were symptoms of brain diseases, could justify *brain and chemical treatments* since that is where the problems were alleged to reside. This has led to a huge industry of finding drug treatments to 'fix' mental health problems, linked to the vague diagnoses, even though this whole logic arises from faulty discourses about 'mental health'.

This has become a huge problem in that: (1) the 'cures' from drug treatments are likely to be little else than distractions and *reducing* life engagement in general ('dumbing down', 'zombifying'); (2) that the drug treatments cause worse changes in behaviour than originally present; and (3) coming off such drug treatments often leads to more problems (Kinderman, 2019; Watson, 2019).

If the 'neurological' problems had actually been located by observing the individual's bad life situations rather than merely in faulty, abstract reasoning, that would be one thing, but given that the 'internal brain disease' reasoning was later used as a discursive justification for drug treatments, the problems have been compounded.

Cognitive behaviour therapy

The last addition was the discursive strategy from academic psychology of using the abstract theories of cognitive psychology to build a 'foundation' to the clinical observations (response 2). The main assumptions here were that people's cognitive processing events go wrong (usually because of some unknown brain disease) and they begin to behave in unusual ways. This is presumed to be a *fault or dysfunction with their cognitive processing* that one day will be identified as a brain disorder. Treatments are then based supposedly on these theoretical notions, although almost all the 'new' techniques of CBT 'deriving from cognitive theory' can be found in Janet's 1919 compendium and before.

Once again, these discursive strategies fit in nicely with neoliberal goals of governance and control in modern society, in that each problem behaviour can be identified (through the DSM) as a problem in producing behaviour brought about by a faulty processing unit (presumably due to a brain problem), which can then be slotted into a standard treatment/solution for ridding the client of those behaviours. This has huge flaws in the reasoning and makes a lot of assumptions that are tenuous at best (V4.8). Anyone in modern society with different behaviour can therefore be diagnosed into a category and given the 'appropriate' treatment. At least that was the dream.

Conclusion

To conclude, I will go back to the beginning. At the end of the 1800s, people started showing new and inexplicable behaviours (Guerin, 2019). These cases were given to medical professionals trained in physiology and medicine who tried to show that the behaviours were 'symptoms' of 'underlying' neurological problems. In the absence of finding any known neurological problems, others started talking about them as 'psychological' problems, which was just another way of saying "we do not know where these are coming from" (Guerin, 2017), or else using everyday (vacuous) descriptions such as "due to insanity". These are exactly the three responses to the Gestalt problem taken by Pathway 1 (V4.1).

What was *not* done was to investigate and observe directly the actual worlds of these people (Pathway 2), except for some minimal progress in showing that they were not due to immediate family problems and showing that in many cases there had sometimes been historical traumatic events before these symptoms appeared. But *the effects of the very new social, cultural, economic, patriarchal, and other contexts of everyday life in modernity were not pursued* even though they inevitably created many of the bad situations people were trying to cope with—the trauma, the abuse, the lack of support from the now ubiquitous stranger relationships, the inability to accomplish much if you have no money, etc. One can only imagine the difference if such cases had been given to contextual experts such as social anthropologists rather than to the medical profession (except that good social anthropologists who could actually do contextual observations did not exist then; cf. Luhrmann & Marrow, 2016).

To make things worse, those trying to control and govern the ever-increasing urban population of strangers were able to use the approaches that had been invented to their advantage. With the modern economic assumptions of individualism and individual responsibility in society, and the neoliberal approach of finding packaged, non-social (V5.1) solutions to all problems, the idea that problem behaviours were caused through *individual* brain problems that could be clearly identified by the DSM 'tool' or 'instrument' (the use of these words speaks volumes), and that there would be a standard treatment model for each that could be successfully applied, must have been very attractive. And still is attractive to those who have no sociological imagination.

And thus this leads us to the current state of how we think about and treat 'mental health'. The problems, however, are as follows:

- No such brain disorders have been found.
- Our treatments are not working well and might just be spontaneous improvements in people's life situations.
- Drug regimes are being imposed by the pharmaceutical companies with a huge marketing and lobbying force, but drugs escape the symptoms and do not cure.
- Our (mostly successful) treatments have not really changed since the beginning of the 1900s except in the abstract theoretical edifices that have been constructed to justify them (Janet, 1919/1925).

• The societal bureaucracies have welcomed such faulty approaches because they fit with the neoliberal ideologies and practices of how to govern modern societies, not because they are working well to help people.

To go back to Volume 4 of this series, what we need to do now is to go back to the Gestalt fork in the road, and follow up Pathway 2, *the social and societal contextual analyses of people who exhibit these 'symptoms'* (Fromene & Guerin, 2014; Fromene, Guerin, & Krieg, 2014; Guerin, 2019; Guerin & Guerin, 2012; Ryan, Guerin, Elmi, & Guerin, 2019). Rather than build more 'internal' models and treatments, *we must find ways to observe people's contexts or lifeworlds, and to change those bad life situations giving rise to the behaviours that are hurting them.* Instead of trying to fix the individual's brain, mind, or cognitive processing, we must fix their bad situations in life or help them to survive and thrive in any bad situations they cannot change.

References

Foucault, M. (1970). *The order of things: An archaeology of the human sciences.* London: Pantheon.

Foucault, M. (2009). *History of madness.* London: Routledge.

Fromene, R., & Guerin, B. (2014). Talking to Australian Indigenous clients with borderline personality disorder labels: Finding the context behind the diagnosis. *Psychological Record, 64*, 569–579.

Fromene, R., Guerin, B., & Krieg, A. (2014). Australian Indigenous clients with a borderline personality disorder diagnosis: A contextual review of the literature. *Psychological Record, 64*, 559–567.

Guerin, B. (2017). *How to rethink mental illness: The human contexts behind the labels.* London: Routledge.

Guerin, B. (2019). What do therapists and clients talk about when they cannot explain behaviours? How Carl Jung avoided analysing a client's environments by inventing theories. *Revista Perspectivas em Anályse Comportamento, 10*, 76–97.

Guerin, B., & Guerin, P. (2012). Re-thinking mental health for indigenous Australian communities: Communities as context for mental health. *Community Development Journal, 47*(4), 555–570.

Horney, K. (1935/1999). *The therapeutic process: Essays and lectures.* London: Yale University Press.

Janet, P. (1919/1925). *Psychological healing: A historical and clinical study.* London: George Allen & Unwin.

Johnstone, L., Boyle, M., Cromby, J., Dillon, J., Harper, D., Kinderman, P., … Read, J. (2018). *The Power Threat Meaning Framework: Towards the identification of patterns in emotional distress, unusual experiences and troubled or troubling behaviour, as an alternative to functional psychiatric diagnosis.* Leicester, UK: British Psychological Society.

Jones, E. (1953). *The life and work of Sigmund Freud. Volume 1: 1856–1900. The formative years and the great discoveries.* New York, NY: Basic Books.

Kinderman, P. (2019). *A manifesto for mental health: Why we need a revolution in mental health care.* London: Palgrave Macmillan.

Luhrmann, T. M., & Marrow, J. (Eds.) (2016). *Our most troubling madness: Case studies in schizophrenia across cultures.* London: University of California Press.

Meyer, A. (1948). *The commonsense psychiatry of Dr. Alfred Meyer.* New York, NY: McGraw-Hill.

Miller, P., & Rose, N. (1994). On therapeutic authority: Psychoanalytical expertise under advanced liberalism. *History of the Human Sciences, 7,* 29–64.

Rose, N. (1999). *Governing the soul: The shaping of the private self* (2nd ed.). London: Free Association Books.

Ryan, J., Guerin, P., Elmi, F. H., & Guerin, B. (2019). What can Somali community talk about mental health tell us about our own? Contextualizing the symptoms of mental health. *International Journal of Migration, Health and Social Care, 15,* 13–24.

Watson, J. (2019). *Drop the disorder: Challenging the culture of psychiatric diagnosis.* London: PCCS Books.

2 Contextualizing 'mental health' behaviours

The ideas of this chapter follow from some recent changes that have occurred in our thinking about mental health, and from turning psychology away from Pathway 1 to Pathway 2 (V4.1). I will not spend too long going over these changes, nor giving all the reasons, justifications, and evidence for them, since you can read about all that elsewhere (see Chapter 1; Guerin, 2017; Johnstone et al., 2018; Kinderman, 2019; Watson, 2019).

Psychology and psychiatry have been dominated since their inception in the late 1800s by using the common-sense way of explaining human behaviour: appealing to something or someone inside of us (Pathway 1). This has gone through the homunculus, psyche, mind, mental processes, consciousness, cognitive processes, will, ego, inner child, self, unconscious, embodied cognitive processes, neural networks, associative networks, and now all sorts of new brain metaphors.

These old explanations are now changing, but this does not imply that all the events and observations themselves were just hocus pocus, nor that the experiences people had of them did not exist or were not real. I treat all those mentioned experiences as real, but I argue that the explanations currently given are not correct, in the sense that there is not some inner 'thing' that can explain what people do. More importantly is that our brains do not originate or create or decide our behaviours and our thinking—they are not agentive. So, we only get correlations.

For example, we certainly have a strong feeling that we are conscious beings, especially when compared to being unconscious (like asleep), but we can actually explain this 'consciousness' in other ways than invoking some internal 'space' (V4.4) and, in any case, we cannot appeal to it when we explain human behaviour. "I went into the city *because* I consciously decided to do this." A tautology. All that is being said in the previous sentence is probably true 'in a sense', but the words are not accurate descriptions of what is taking place nor how we should explain this 'going into the city' (see V4 for more arguments).

The new contextual version for understanding people

In brief, our behaviour arises directly from and is shaped by our interactions with our environments or lifeworlds. This is just as true for those actions, talking, and thinking currently labelled 'mental health', as for any others. I will use the phrases 'lifeworld' or 'context' sometimes because 'environment' is often treated in psychology as just the physical environment, whereas here I am meaning all the observable and not easily observable societal structures around us, not just the physical environment. Just as we cannot walk through walls, we also cannot go and just get $1,000,000 out of our bank account if it is not in there, nor smash patriarchy overnight to improve life for women and men. These societal contexts all structure our worlds and shape our behaviours (V5.3).

I will give more details about these 'environments' in the next chapter, but they include all the parts of the world that shape our actions, talking, and thinking, and that can facilitate or hinder what we do, including:

- social relationships (which includes language use)
- economics in a broad sense (what we have to do to get things in order to live)
- patriarchy
- history
- cultural practices
- opportunities
- colonization

I also frequently refer to 'social context' because 99 per cent of what shapes us only works through other people, whether family or strangers. So, they amount to the same, but when talking about some topics, especially language and economics, it is good to remind ourselves that these are shaped by *social* contexts, not any other parts of the world. I contend that a lot of the misdirection of Western philosophy and psychology over the last few hundred years has arisen because it was forgotten that both words and money only work at all through people—they are both social. Thinking they arise all by themselves or as part of a 'natural' world, has messed these disciplines up (V5.2)!

So, to understand what people do, we must know *all* the environments or contexts that shape their behaviours, and those contexts could be part of any or all the above (V2; V5.3).

Applying this to mental health

If we apply this to the behaviours seen as 'mental health' issues, the point is that they do not arise from a brain disease, lesion, or chemical imbalance, as the medical models say. Nor do life conflicts and stress lead to brain diseases, lesions, or chemical imbalances, as the stress-mental health models would have us believe. And they do not arise from some 'inner' (totally metaphorical) world of mind or psyche.

The most dificult part of this for readers is to *stop thinking of these behaviours as tied to or even as associated together in groups by some inner brain disease.* There are two parts that need drastic rethinking, therefore:

- Mental health behaviours *originate* from an 'inner' cause.
- Several 'problem' behaviours *go together* somehow because of this same 'inner' disease.

My goal is to try and show how the 'mental health' behaviours directly originate from the bad situations in people's lives, and that they are shaped separately. If two behaviours (including talking and thinking) *are* commonly observed together, this is because the person's bad situations originate both, not because there is a disease that links them. Figure 2.1 is the current psychiatric way of thinking for a single diagnosis of 'schizophrenia spectrum'.

This is sometimes replaced by stress-health models of different sorts but they follow this same logic or thinking, except that 'environmental factors' lead to the brain diseases and the rest is the same (see Figure 2.2).

Some more recent models of mental health disagree with the brain disease part (there has never been any evidence for this) but basically see the DSM groupings as okay, so in their logic or thinking the 'symptoms' still form a group (see Figure 2.3)

But the social contextual logic or thinking pulls this further apart by getting rid of the groupings altogether from the DSM. Bad life situations directly shape the individual behaviours that are observed and experienced and that cause distress (and, as we will see later, a lot of other behaviours that 'mental health' experts usually ignore). If a few of these behaviours/ symptoms are found by observation to group together frequently, that is

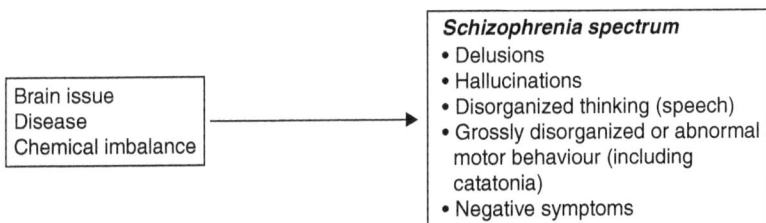

Figure 2.1 Current psychiatric (DSM) model of 'symptoms' arising from brain diseases

Schizophrenia spectrum
• Delusions
• Hallucinations
• Disorganized thinking (speech)
• Grossly disorganized or abnormal motor behaviour (including catatonia)
• Negative symptoms

Bad life events Stress Inability to cope	→	'Predisposition' to mental disease	→	Brain issue Disease Chemical imbalance

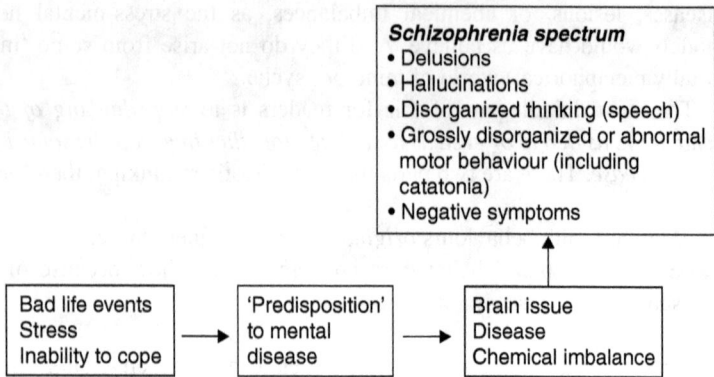

Figure 2.2 Current life event stress models of mental health

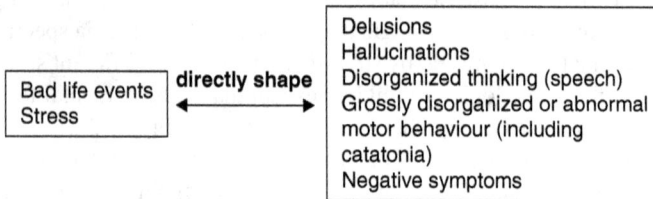

Bad life events Stress	**directly shape** ←→	Delusions Hallucinations Disorganized thinking (speech) Grossly disorganized or abnormal motor behaviour (including catatonia) Negative symptoms

Figure 2.3 Some recent models that see the 'mental health' issues arising from bad life events, but the DSM groupings of symptoms remain

because *the bad situation tends to shape them together*, not because a brain disease is somehow causing them all simultaneously. Further, if there is a 'predisposition' (whatever that means) then that is also *in* the bad situations; your life opportunities and barriers have made it likely that you will be placed into such bad situations (see Figure 2.4).

So, the behaviours and thoughts seen in 'mental health' issues are shaped directly by *bad life situations and conflicts* just as any other behaviours and thoughts are shaped by our lifeworlds (V4). They are ways of *adapting* to change or survive bad situations, or else trying to *escape* those bad situations. Such behaviours and thoughts might have been functional in their original form, but have become *exaggerated, locked into* the bad situations, and *alternative behaviours have become blocked* (Guerin, 2017). For the worst cases, the behaviours are obviously not working to change the person's bad social environments, but they are locked in, difficult to change, and with few alternatives possible.

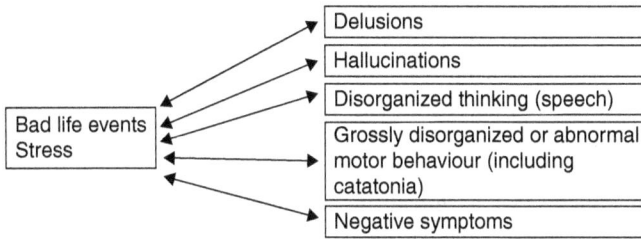

Figure 2.4 The 'mental health' model of this book in which individual symptoms arise from unique bad life events and can be shaped independently

More behaviours are shaped by bad life situations than just the 'mental health' behaviours

The ways of surviving or escaping bad situations not only include 'mental health' behaviours, but also the uses of violence, 'criminal' activities, excessive or dependent drug use, leaving the situation and social relationships altogether and starting again, becoming alternative, exploitation of other people, or just 'putting up with it', even if not happy (Woodiwiss, 1950).

This raises the question of why the 'mental health' behaviours are even seen as a special group? Why are they not seen as just more in a series of behaviours that are commonly shaped when trying to live in untenable conditions—and no different in principle to using crime to escape your bad situation, or walking out and starting again? In fact, some behaviours shaped to 'escape' bad conditions have always been 'borderline' as to whether they really are 'mental health' behaviours and the difference has been confusing: are violence, gambling, and excessive or dependent drug taking 'mental health' issues? If not then why not?

The behaviours and thoughts seen in 'mental health' issues do have some special properties, but contextually they are not in principle any different from our other 'normal' behaviours and thoughts (Guerin, 2017). Their special properties include the following:

- The environments that have shaped the 'mental health' behaviours are not easy to observe.
- Alternative behaviours are blocked so it is not easy to see why these behaviours were shaped instead of ones that might be expected in 'normal' circumstances to help change the bad situation.
- The behaviours can become chronic if they get locked into these bad situations.

- If chronic, the behaviours can become exaggerated (to try to have a new effect on changing things) and it is even less easy to see their original function in the person's life to change the situation.
- The behaviours themselves might not be related to any immediate functioning if the situation is really bad, so they might not 'make sense' to casual observers (including 50-minute conversations with a therapist).

To put this bluntly, we have bad life situations (see Chapter 3) that shape many dysfunctional, conflictual, and stressful behaviours and thoughts (see Chapter 4), and lead to real pain and suffering. For some of these attempts to deal with, cope with, or escape the bad situations:

- They are 'successful' and the bad situation is escaped or avoided.
- We ignore them and our circumstances change in some other way.
- They arise from more obviously bad situations and are referred to professionals other than psychologists (police, social workers, financial advisors, etc.).
- They are seen as 'criminal' and dealt with separately by police.
- The environment/lifeworld that is shaping the behaviours cannot be easily observed (because of external context not because they are hidden 'within' the person) and they get labelled as 'mental health' issues.

So, escaping a life of poverty and abuse by using violence or criminal activities will be dealt with by police because the issue *appears* obvious (you steal to get money, don't you?). But when a child lives with a seemingly 'good' middle-class family but starts to hear voices, there is no obvious or 'explainable' source for this so they will be labelled as having a 'mental' or 'psychological' problem and sent to psychiatrists and psychologists (just as we saw in Chapter 1 for the late 1800s). These behaviours shaped by bad situations are then automatically attributed to something inside the person or in their head (Pathway 1), or to 'spirits' and other similar reasons. We use the same reasoning when we are talking about 'misbehaving' animals and cars (see Figure 2.5).

To give two examples: first, if someone was to start a fight with you in a public place and hit you, it would be clear as to what is shaping your subsequent anger and any retaliatory behaviour and you would have to explain to the police or law courts what happened. If you were to start exhibiting that same anger and retaliatory behaviour with random strangers then 'mental health' questions would be asked, and the professional discourses would be about 'something within you' driving your bizarre actions and 'aggressive impulses'.

As a second example, in the nineteenth and twentieth centuries in Western countries, society's greater opportunities for males (patriarchy) was

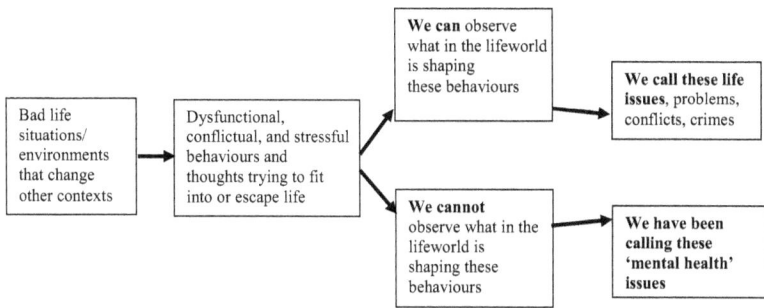

Figure 2.5 Our attributions of how behaviours arise from our bad life situations depend on whether or not we can easily see those life contexts, which in turn depends on the effort put into observing and analysing someone's life situations

enacted through societal power legally given to the father of a household. For women (wives or daughters), their lack of opportunities and restrictions in life had an easily observable 'target' in the husband or father, so the dysfunction, pain, and stress from this for women was not a 'mental health' issue (even though the 'power' of men was ordained through legal and other societal systems). Instead, it was seen as a more direct issue about control within the family, which could still be taken to the courts although women would rarely gain any control this way. Such issues of 'problem daughters and wives' would be dealt with by the father and his legal power, church members, restricting the women even further, or ostracism in the extreme case ("Get thee to a nunnery!").

But in our current Western societies, fathers no longer have such power because capitalism has brought about a society almost fully built on stranger or contractual relationships, and children can now more easily function independently outside of the family. There is still a strong patriarchy operating, however, but for most contemporary women these patriarchal limits on their behaviour are now enacted by strangers and bureaucracies rather than by their husband or father per se. This has meant that the reactive behaviours, pain, conflicts, and stress over reduced life opportunities now have *no easily observable* source of shaping—because it is embedded in the history and creation of capitalist and neoliberal social structures. What this has meant is that from the time a little before Freud and ever since, women have been referred to 'mental health' services (which we saw in Chapter 1 were probably created for this change in societal relationships in the first place) because *no easily observable source* could be found that might have shaped their 'unusual' behaviours called 'hysteria' (Guerin, 2017). And the male medical personnel running the 'clinics' and 'asylums' were also oblivious to the new and hidden forms of *societal enacted patriarchy* (Guerin, 2019).

Overall, the ways in which 'not easily observed' environments affect our judgements has dire consequences for our discourses and decisions about what is 'mental health' and how to help. It means that whether or not some behaviours and thoughts are talked about as part of a 'mental illness' completely depends upon arbitrary criteria such as (1) *what is salient* in any context and (2) *how much time and energy you bother to spend* in finding out those contexts. In lieu of actually observing clients *in situ*, a frequent substitute marker is whether or not the behaviours and thoughts disrupt the 'normal functioning' of their lives, which requires less effort.

So, any behaviours and thoughts might be labelled as a 'mental illness' if the following apply:

- The contextual problems giving rise to the suffering are not clear in normal life.
- The contextual problems giving rise to the suffering are hidden in some way.
- The contextual problems giving rise to the suffering disrupt our life so we do not function in the normal way (and what is 'normal' keeps changing).
- The suffering from the contextual problems disrupts our life.
- There are multiple social relationships or resources, but they are contradictory or conflicting as they are:
  - balanced evenly;
  - mutually exclusive with punishments attached for doing the opposite;
  - long-term versus short-term conflicts.
- Contexts cascade for other reasons and become a social trap.
- Someone outside sees our behaviour and does not understand the contexts operating.
- The professionals do not spend time observing the person's multiple contexts and certainly not *in situ*.

So, people do not *have* mental health issues; they have bad and conflictual life situations of many sorts that lead to issues and stress in their lives, but … if the sources of these conflicts cannot easily be seen or named, then they are more likely to be referred to as 'mental health' issues or 'psychological' problems.

If it is not obvious what has shaped the behaviours and thoughts, then we attribute this to a 'mental illness' (Pathway 1 logic), and if not, it is a normal life issue, albeit still bad and leading to suffering. In the first case we might be referred to a psychologist or psychiatrist, in the second case we might be referred to social workers, police, financial advisors, life coaches, or a pastoral care person. Even surviving bad situations through violence, 'criminal' activities, excessive or dependent drug use, lying, and deceiving have always been ambiguous with respect to 'mental health' ("Mad or bad?"; Geyer, 2008; Woodiwiss, 1950). My argument is that where a 'cause' is obvious, they are not considered 'mental health' issues; but where a 'cause' is not obvious, they are. But in between there is no strict and fast division. We need to study them together and work on changing the bad situations together (see Chapter 5).

The worst problem with all this is that it all *depends on your ability and effort to find out the life contexts for someone with 'problematic' behaviour,* and this has nothing to do with the actual behaviours and suffering we are dealing with. It is almost arbitrary, relying on how much the professional knows about life situations, their training, how much time they are allowed, and what they choose to observe. The distinction between what has been called 'psychological' issues and the other bad life issues *only depends* on whether the contexts that have given rise to the issues can be easily observed. And of huge importance, this also means *the people in bad situations themselves are not likely to know where their behaviours have arisen from as well.*

And as pointed out by others (e.g. Rose, 1962), psychologists, psychiatrists, and philosophers (in the very early days) were possibly *the worst people* to deal with such issues because they had poor training in contextual observation and analysis, especially those coming from the medical profession where internal diseases are the focus for all causality. Anthropologists are far better trained in contextual observations, contextual analysis, and contextual questioning, along with detectives, some sociologists, and some community psychologists.

To make this more explicit, there are many non-obvious ways in which the contexts or causes for behaviour can be hidden, thus leading to a false attribution of a 'mental health' cause, but most of these have nothing directly to do with the behaviour itself or causes. For example:

• You have not spent enough time observing all the person's behaviours and actions; even if you have good reasons for this—it takes too long, your boss will not allow extra time, your research needs to finish quickly. In each case you will still miss what is going wrong and have to resort to averages or abstract theorizing.
• You have not spent enough time observing in context.
• There are historical events and contexts that you have not observed or have not thought to find out about.

- You have little or no lived experience yourself in the actual bad life situations a person is going through, so you are oblivious to their real situation.
- There is something that the person has successfully avoided or escaped from in the past by doing what they are doing (the 'mental health' behaviours), and you cannot observe that outcome because it does not actually occur anymore since it is being successfully escaped or avoided.
- There are key elements of the context for behaviour that are not present in the *current* situation (including your office), so you cannot see them.
- There are key elements of the context for behaviour that the person has kept secret or is hiding for other contextual reasons that you also do not know about.
- There are key elements of the context for behaviour that simply do not fit into (your) ordinary experience and so these are not observed even though they potentially could be.
- The behaviours work well because the contexts are not obvious; even for 'normal' behaviours it is often best to not know the contexts in which someone's behaviour towards you arises.
- Where language use (including thinking) is prevalent in a context, because the social control of language is frequently difficult to observe without a lot of effort (because the words distract us from what is really going on in conversation—social negotiation).
- Where the bad situations arise from societal control and limitations these cannot often be observed easily (the effects of capitalism, bureaucracy, modern patriarchy; see V5.3)

The upshot is that correcting this is not easy (Watson, 2019), and the *research methods* of psychology and psychiatry have not been useful for discovering and describing the contexts from which our actions, talking, and thinking arise (see V5.9, Table 9.1). Social anthropology, some sociology, and community psychology have much better research and intervention methods for gleaning the contexts of people's lives, but they require more time and engagement than sitting in an office and chatting to someone for 50 minutes (Guerin, 2018; Guerin, Leugi, & Thain, 2018). To a person from Mars it might seem that understanding mental health has been a very *lazy* business, with fictitious internal states being set up as the 'explanations' in lieu of any real effort put into finding out about the person's actual lifeworld outside of the therapist's office (Guerin, 2019).

Before going on to consider thinking and 'mental health' in context, Box 2.1 includes an exercise to help you break from attributing everything people do to 'internal' causes. See how well this works for you!

Box 2.1 Practical exercise to experience how while we may seem to be controlled from inside of us, the external contexts are actually originating what we do, say, and think

- Go into a park on a windy day where there are some big trees.
- Watch a tree for a while but try to imagine that the wind is not real—there is no wind in the context really.
- *Instead*, imagine that the tree itself is moving its own branches and leaves (like an Ent in *The Lord of the Rings*).
- You could imagine that the tree is waving at you, doing a tree sign language, or dancing for you.
- It all originates from inside the tree.
- It is a biological event, originating from inside the tree's cells, or maybe the tree has some neural structures or cognitive architecture?
- You should be able to do it; it is not hard to imagine that the tree is moving itself.
- It is easier to do this if you remove yourself from the context of the wind. Try sitting inside a car with the windows up, for example, or watch from inside your house.
- And once this works for you, it will seem that the *only* way to stop the tree from moving is to disable or dumb down its internal cellular activity; inject some cellulose-inhibiting drugs; that will stop it.

The messages to learn from this are as follows:

- It is not difficult to ignore the external contexts (the wind) and then imagine that the tree is waving at you all by itself, and that this is caused by its internal cell structures or 'tree cognition'; it is easy to do, and it begins to seem real.
- However, *in fact*, the external wind is making the tree move.
- Even so, the biological cells of the tree are still involved as they bend; but they are just not the *origin* of the behaviour.
- The origins of the behaviour are not *in* the tree but in the contexts—the wind in this case.
- *The less you can see or participate in these contexts, the easier* it becomes to imagine that it is all originating from inside the tree.
- And actually, the only *real* way to stop the behaviour is to change the contexts; stop the wind by placing windbreaks around the

tree, support the tree in its windy context by stopping the strong winds blowing it around.

The messages to learn about medical models of mental health:

* This is actually how the medical models of 'mental health' work.
* All 'problem' behaviours are imagined to be originating *inside* the person in their biology (despite no evidence).
* If you ignore the person's bad life situations (their contexts), it is really easy to imagine these internal models as real.
* But you should not participate in or observe the person's real-life situations because you will begin to doubt that it all originates inside the person (so stay in your office, talk to them away from their contexts, don't build a relationship with them, keep the windows up!).
* However, *in fact*, the 'mental health' behaviours originate in people's bad life situations; your clients are trying to survive with hurricanes blowing through their worlds and nothing is helping as their behaviours get more extreme from the stronger winds.
* And yes, the brain is still involved, but not as the *origin* of these behaviours.
* And yes, if you bother to go into and observe their real-life bad situations, their behaviour begins to make sense ("What has happened to you?", "What bad winds are blowing through your existence so that whatever you do does not seem to make things better for you?").
* And to help them, you need to change the person's bad life situations; that should be the focus of any intervention or change, not altering their brain or chemistry.

Contextualizing thinking and perceiving for 'mental health'

I am adding extra here on thinking and perceiving because they are important when contextualizing 'mental health'. This is not because they are easily affected by brain diseases but because they fit most of the criteria given earlier for what is even included as 'mental health' or not in the first place. They are also prevalent in human life so they are always available as behaviours that can be shaped in new ways when in bad situations so as to try and change those situations—when other behaviours are blocked or not possible.

The idea is that the so-called 'thought disorders' are just extreme variations on 'normal' talking, thinking (V4.4), and imaging (V4.5), which are shaped from being in bad situations with few alternative opportunities to change anything. Because talking and thinking are such a large part of our lives now, a large part of the DSM is therefore about talking and thinking shaped in new ways (see Chapter 4). For this reason, it is worthwhile going over some of the analyses of talking and thinking, and a bit on imaging ('hallucinations' and hearing voices).

Alternative variations on 'thinking' and 'thought disorders'

In V4.4, I outlined how we can think and talk about thinking in new ways: that thinking is the same as talking and responding to people's talk but not said out loud. This means that it is controlled externally to us and it consists of bits of all our conversations, discourses, texts, etc., which shape us both to talk out loud and to think. Our brains do not *originate* our thoughts. Like other language forms, thoughts have been shaped by our dealings and social negotiations with people in our language or discursive communities. It is like we live in a fish tank of many discourses, which we take in and regurgitate as our social groupings change, but we hardly notice and so think they originate inside of us.

This change in thinking can be both deflating and exhilarating. For many, the idea that *we* (whoever that is) do not originate our thoughts seems like an attack on their personhood and integrity. It seems like we would no longer have control or that you, as a person, are no longer important. While true in a way, this is not as bad as it sounds. Your personhood and its integrity (Scalabrini, Mucci, Esposito, Damiani & Northoff, 2020) are about the environments in which you have been embedded and what you have done (including what you say and think), and we each have a remarkable history of these, which is unique to each of us and important. Your real self is your exchanges—actions and talking—with all your social relationships, the environment around you, and the social systems in which we are embedded, not just a story you make up about yourself (V5.5).

Further, a bad thing is that whenever something is said to be 'internal' to us, it allows blaming the victim for something that was really shaped in our worlds, not by some internal 'I' thing. For some years, therapists working with people who were given labels of 'dysfunctional thinking' have been trying to get across the idea that they are not responsible for their bad thoughts, they do not have to 'own' them or take responsibility as the creators of these thoughts (except legally). These thought patterns are nonetheless still painful and hurting for such people and those around them, and it is the discursive environments which need to be changed.

Therefore, I wish to examine a number of experiences in which 'normal' thinking, as we mostly assume it, is disrupted or changed (by the external contexts changing), and try to think through what might be going on in such cases if the shaping of our thoughts is treated as external (cf. Reed, 1974, who does this via Pathway 1). These are not final answers or complete explanations, but suggestions for further exploration (Scalabrini, Mucci, Esposito, Damiani & Northoff, 2020). One beneficial outcome of treating thoughts as being shaped externally is that they become potentially observable, in the sense that you can in theory trace *who* or *which social or cultural contexts* shaped those discourses as thoughts, and then identify what can be changed in those relationships to change the thoughts if they are causing problems.

I will not cover all of the clinical or 'dysfunctional' varieties of thinking, Chapter 4 will look at those more closely, although I will suggest analyses for some of them here. But it is really important to get the idea that thinking is shaped out there in our discursive worlds and so many 'normal' ideas are very wrong, including: that we only have one thought or 'voice' at all times, that voice is 'me', and I do what that voice says because it is me. This allows that all sorts of other experiences with thinking—labelled by psychiatrists as dissociative, hearing voices, hallucinations, etc.—are very real but they do not originate in your head. Such thought experiences can be treated in new ways and handled more respectfully than they have been in the past when called 'dysfunctional thinking', 'disordered thoughts', or 'thoughts disorders'.

Traditional views of thinking

The traditional view of thinking is that of 'processes' going on inside the head that *originate* internally even though the original 'input' was actually from outside the person. We generally have a thread of thinking going on inside us (in fact we are responding to external events with language but not out loud) that correlates with, and is usually said to control directly, what we do. This thread of thinking is thought of in some sense as our 'self' or 'ego', and we then believe (wrongly) that speech or writing are used to express or communicate these 'inner' thoughts to other people in the world outside (whereas I suggest that we are saying them to do things to people and they originated 'out there' in the first place).

Thinking is also traditionally linked to problem solving, in the sense of seeming to produce new solutions without any immediate change in the environment. The environment seems to stay static and yet with some 'internal' thinking we can say (usually) a new solution. This was partially supported by the claims of the cognitive revolution that we can do things without environmental 'input' and construct the world inside our heads (but see V4.1).

Finally, the term 'thinking' is also traditionally used for *any* processes going on which seem to have no sensory input determining them. If I am daydreaming there seems to be 'events happening inside me' that are not determined by sensory input, and these are also occasionally called 'thinking' even though they involve events more related to seeing than to talking. If you are daydreaming and someone asks you what you are doing, you might reply, "Just thinking about things".

Before considering some varieties of thinking it is useful to revise how the current view differs from the previous traditional views (cf. Ryle, 1971). Thinking is a broad term and other responses that do not occur are sometimes also referred to as thinking, as we saw for daydreaming. The main thing seems to be that we have multiple responses in any context, but we cannot do them all. In some contexts, these (the ones not actually enacted) are still responses and seem to affect us, and they are often called thinking. It so happens that because our most frequent, learned behaviour in any context is to *say* something, thinking will consist of a disproportionate number of language responses, more than talking itself.

Contextualizing some experiences of variations from 'normal' thinking

In this section I will go through some of the diverse experiences of 'thinking' and how they can be mapped contextually. None of them are 'pathological' although they currently can get diagnostic labels if they arise from a bad life situation and cannot get changed easily. If the contextual view of language use and thinking is on the right path, then they are just contextual variations on 'normal' or 'status quo' ways we are supposed to talk, not a disease. However, if they occur when a person is in a bad situation (see Chapter 3) and is suffering, then we need to look at how that bad context is affecting and changing their thinking—and then changing those environments is what is important, not pathologizing an experience as if it was a disease the person *has*.

These experiences of variations in 'normal' thinking and imaging also occur in pleasant or interesting situations of life, in new or challenging situations, when intoxicated or using drugs, or even with lack of sleep or severe hunger. Sometimes they are just short-lived, when something out of the ordinary happens and passes quickly. Some last longer and are just 'put up with' (see Chapter 3) through life, and others get integrated as regular but sometimes odd (to other people that is) parts of someone's life. Most people have some foibles, quirks, and eccentricities that people accept, or they are not spoken of.

1. *The main experience of what we call thinking is just our talking responses (and other responses) but not made out loud.* Not being said

out loud gives thinking slightly different properties to talking out loud
(V4.4), but thinking is engaged with our worlds and resource–social
relationships pathways, just like our talking. Thinking therefore will
be made up of sentences, phrases, and other conversational snippets,
things we might say rather than single words.

2.   *We always have multiple language responses in any situation, most of
     which are not said out loud.* Our experience is that one of these seems
     'clearer' (even though not said out loud). This is variously called our
     consciousness, 'me voice', 'critical voice', or 'command voice' (V5.5).
     It is sometimes called our 'me voice' because we assume this is our
     'self' speaking to ourselves (which is not a good description of what
     is happening). It is called the 'critical voice' sometimes because in
     modern society at least, our immediate reactions to anything is to give
     oppositional, competitive, or critical responses but these frequently are
     not said out loud. It is sometimes called the 'command voice' because
     as we are doing things in life we often have simultaneous descriptions
     of what we are doing or might do, and the experience (wrongly) is that
     we 'give ourselves' commands and then follow them (in reality the
     simultaneous dialogue is for other people if needed later). V4.4 has
     more on this. Which talking is the 'me', critical, or command voice
     arises from the situations you are in, not from some decision made
     inside you. When something bad happens unexpectedly and you cannot
     talk out loud, this bad event will likely be the focus of this voice.

3.   From the above, *some experiences of anxiety occur when we cannot,
     for many reasons, have this simultaneous 'me' responding about what
     we are doing.* This is consequential for people if they are in punishing
     or highly critical worlds and constantly need to justify or explain why
     they are doing what they are doing (or going to do). It is as if we auto-
     matically assume that if you cannot say what you are doing and why,
     then the situation is bad! Always be ready to explain yourself!

4.   *Our discourses, voices, thinking, and talking are always shaped by
     people* (abstract like the media, or real like an earlier argument you had
     with a friend that day), which means the thoughts that 'pop into our head'
     come from our community and social conversations and arguments. This
     means our thoughts are always shaped by others and do not originate
     inside us. But our normal experience is of the opposite, that our thoughts
     are 'us' and that they control what we do (see more in V5.6).

     But in some special contexts (such as reading a good book or
     watching a good movie), we lose that experience and our words start to
     seem foreign to us, as if planted there, and we are not in control. When
     these experiences get tangled up in bad situations in life, they currently
     are called pathological, although for examples like reading they are

clearly not. As mentioned above, the bad situations some people are in when these experiences arise might be labelled 'pathological', but not the experiences themselves. Titchener used to get this experience with students by having them repeat a word or phrase over and over, and experience how the word 'loses meaning'.

5. Because our thoughts are shaped by our discursive communities and are there to do things to people and not to be representations of the world, *there is no truth or falsity that can be applied to words, including thoughts*. Our language does not have the property of being true or false, it is just a behaviour we have learned to affect people (Guerin, 2016). We can say anything, in other words, and the only analysis is *what it does to people, not whether it is true or false*.

6. Even though most of our experience seems to be that we construct our thoughts ourselves, *for contextualizing all talk and thinking we need to consider the social contexts* (audiences) that shaped those thoughts around the social relationship issues. Again, people sometimes do experience this when their thinking seems to get 'dissociated' or 'detached' from 'reality'. They *lose* that normal (but false) experience we have that thinking (1) is a singular strand, (2) controls our behaviour, and (3) is originated by a 'me'. We appear to have these properties normally because our social worlds are typically rigid and stable, not because they are a true reflection of some 'inner world'. *The 'dissociative' world is closer to the contextual idea in fact*: our words and thinking do not control our behaviour (Scalabrini, Mucci, Esposito, Damiani & Northoff, 2020).

The 'dissociated' experiences arising from variations being shaped in any of the three ways above, make it seem as if the thoughts become disembodied from 'yourself' (which ironically I see as a true reflection of events—thoughts originate outside of us). This dissociation will usually be treated as pathological if it is extensive, but it reflects the reality, I believe—our thoughts do not originate inside us and are not controlled by 'us'. If the experience continues, the real 'mental health' question is: how did this experience arise from the person's worlds (bad situations usually; see Chapter 3) such that they were not able to maintain the normal pattern? The normal experience is status quo but if you do not 'fit into' life, because of your bad situations, the status quo can vary. You are not pathological, but your situation probably is. (The answer? *Fix the situation not the person*)

So, ironically, our normal state of affairs with respect to thinking and control of our behaviour (single stream of thought, thinking controls our behaviour, an internal 'me' originates our thoughts), only appears that way because we typically have stable and limited social worlds wrapped around us. Variations often appear in everyday life, but they are not talked about. When the variations are extreme, because of extreme life situations, the shaping cannot easily be seen so they are mistakenly attributed to something going wrong 'inside us' with our 'normal' thinking.

7. With respect to rethinking imagery contextually (V4.5), a key point that differs from the traditional views of psychology is that *we do not see with sensations*. As Gibson made clear (V4.5), we move around the world by responding directly to *changes* on the retina and other sensory events, we do not 'take in' anything of this to 'process'. At the same time, however, just as language use becomes thinking when not out loud, *we have strong experiences in which it seems like we can see things we have previously seen when there is nothing in front of us.*

These experiences are called various names such as imagery, hallucinations, images, and sometimes thinking. However, unlike language thinking, which is mostly experienced as coming from 'inside' us, the experiences of imagery and hallucinations are some-times like they are occurring outside of us, but other times they are like thinking (language use) and the experience is that we see them as if somewhere 'inside' of us. Hearing music constantly, for example, seems like the latter—that it is going on 'inside you'. Hearing voices, on the other hand, often has the experience of voices coming from outside you. Once again, which it is depends on how easy it is to observe the external shaping.

So, images are clearly related to past changes learned in our sensory systems, but they are the result of some special external conditions and not the result of moving about the world (e.g. Guerin, 1990, V4.5). When there are external conditions present (someone saying to you, "Can you picture your mother's face?"), we are *somehow* able to have the same or similar perceptual responses reoccur that occurred when there really was an object in front of us. But it is important to remember that they are not generated in, or do not originate, in our brains or some 'internal processors'. Like language-based thinking, images occur as events when there are external contexts in place; they are events, not objects or pictures.

In some cases, people report having imagery, but they are experien-cing language use and discourses *about* what seems to be imagery. That is, they are re-responding with words and people previously *talking* about their mother's face, not re-responding with similar perceptual responses to the original direct perception. "Yes, and I remember they always said her red hair was amazing", rather than, "Yes, I can picture her red hair clearly, as if in front of me now!"

Gibson also pointed out, just as thinking is talking not said out loud, that such imagery has a few different properties from direct perception, but these only happen because the perceptual responses occur without anything changing on the retina, not because they are new or different perceptual responses. For example, *we cannot explore images* in the way we can (visually) explore real objects when we see them (see Chapter 5). We also cannot touch them or use our other senses to explore them. They also require special contexts to be in place for them to occur, especially with regards to the proximate environment. Such special properties that differ from normal 'direct perception', have been described for 'seeing' hallucinations, movies, photographs, and art (Deleuze, 1986, 1989; Gibson, 1971, 1978, 1979). They could be utilized for working with people who hallucinate.

8. *Many of the strange experiences of perception are actually to do with language problems.* One of the main outcomes of direct perception is social and discursive responding such as 'naming' (V.5). We see and name things and events around us, even if we do not see them fully. Most times when there are 'visual illusions', the confusion is a language problem—the full context for seeing (optical array) has been stripped of all textual detail and so we *cannot* give more definitive names. The language responses are usually even prompted externally: "What do you see? A vase or two faces?" Gibson did not use illusions for research because there was no point in studying how environmental textures and contextual variations changed direct perception when you have stripped away all the context in the first place! It does not tell us anything useful.

9. In a similar way to the above, *other senses can allow us to behave in the same way, including sounds and kinaesthetic sensations.* All these could also be called 'thinking'. We can 'hear' music when none is playing (à la language responding or perceptual responding), and we can 'feel' things on our skin when nothing is there. Again, these are not originating 'inside of us' but are the same perceptual response events as occurred when things *were* in front of us, but without them being there (just as we can talk as if to a friend when the friend is not there, but there are differences). So, thinking as 'talking but not out loud' is equivalent to imagery as 'our same perceptual responses reoccurring when nothing is there'. The sounds or feelings arise from some other external contexts (such as being asked, "Can you hear the 'Stairway to Heaven'" opening riff in your head?" or hearing the first part of some music played).

10. *All the language, visual perception, sound, and kinaesthetic forms of 'thinking', need to be learned.* We know very little about how these

forms of responding arise and from what contexts when growing up. This is partly because psychology, as for everyday theories, treat them as spontaneously arising from within us as part of a 'self', so they must be hereditary or special abilities. We still need to find out more, and how they can be trained in as adults.

Many people do not 'see' (or 'think') imagery or sounds very easily, so how are they trained? Clearly, the first thing is for the person to spend a lot of time using perceptual and auditory perception, and experiencing these perceptual responses directly first, and to excess (overlearn). If you want to learn to hear 'music in your head' you need to listen to a lot of music first! In other words, start overlearning sonic perceptual responding. This is the same as the 'overlearning' of language that the majority of people go through in childhood and beyond (V4.3). The overuse of language in our lives makes the 'language-use thinking' more prevalent (and wrongly seem already built-in) than the 'perceptual and auditory-use thinking'. I have met some people, however, who can only 'think' by saying things out loud. So, if we overlearn auditory or visual (perceptual) responses, this seems to afford us rehearing sounds and images when they are not being played out loud. You can learn to hear music when none is playing.

11. *It is often difficult to distinguish between word-events and non-word-events in everyday life* (V4.3). The first are shaped and maintained by the effects on people whereas the second is not. If the words are said out loud, this is usually clear. For example, if I say, "I really like chocolate", this is a social word event and not directly related to the physical chocolate, since my action (talking) does not affect any chocolate, only people. But because 'thinking' is not out loud, this difference becomes much more difficult to distinguish. That is, *things can appear less real and more imaginary when thought rather than when spoken out loud.* So for studying thinking it is important to analyse the conditions that shaped that talking not being out loud (V4.4), and for studying imagery it is important to study what contexts facilitate someone re-responding with the same perceptual responses when nothing is there (V4.5). These two points will be important in Chapter 4 when understanding 'thought disorders'.

12. *When we stop responding out loud with our 'normal' verbal responses to things and events, this is often called 'internalization'.* Rather than something having gone 'inside the head', internalization needs to be thought of as more like talking without saying things out loud. The responding still arises from the external contexts of the person, and *it is the external conditions for not speaking out loud* that lead to 'internalizing' and that need investigating (see V4.4, Box 4.1). If 'internalizing'

is a problem for someone's life, then the real problems are the external contexts that stopped, punished, or prevented the responding out loud (see V4.3). Just getting the person to say whatever has been 'internalized' out loud will not always succeed, therefore, if the social punishing conditions are still there.

13. *Hearing voices* is again an experience known for millennia, which can be present in everyday life and useful, but if the person is already in bad life situations they cannot change, it can lead to suffering. Contextually, any and all of our thoughts are really 'hearing voices', but they usually do not appear to come from outside us. Our thoughts are parts of our conversational responding and other social discourses that are shaped externally, so really they are 'voices outside of us'. Only some people can 'hear' them by re-responding with auditory perceptual responses.

In everyday experience, our thoughts are like voices coming from outside of us (from our social life of discourses) but at least in the Western world, we have learned to think of them as originating inside us. The so-called 'pathological' instances of voice hearing are different. They originate in bad situations in life, and the shaping of thoughts no longer fits into the simple 'me' voice that controls 'me' doing what I do. What would be 'me thoughts' normally give a different experience in bad situations because the social contexts are messed up: opposing and contradictory social audiences, messed-up social relationships, messed-up cultural relationships, and the modern influence of the 'generalized other' voice from societal contexts that pressures us. The result is the experience of thoughts appearing as real voices (and some join with strong imagery to really give the experience of people actually speaking outside of you) and this leads to problems thinking about the control of our behaviour by thoughts (which does not happen anyway, but that is our prevailing everyday experience, V5.6).

So, imagine that all of your many and sometimes opposing thoughts you normally have in different situations you now experience as different people talking to you as if externally, and your 'me' voice becomes a minor character (this is scary for most people). In fact, it has been described like a theatre, with each of your many thoughts being a different character in a play. Now, if life was simple and straightforward then this might not be a problem. But this experience is usually only noticed when the social controls over thinking are messed up, so life spirals out of control with complex situations and hence a lot of the thoughts (characters) are in conflict. Imagine your usual 'me voice' commentary now seeming like it is coming from another person, all your verbal commentaries and preparing excuses out of 'your' (me voice) control! Scary …

As all those who work for voice hearers' groups know, the trick is not to stop the voices (they are just complex and different thoughts like we all have) but to *manage* them better within the bad life situations while trying to change those situations (Longden, Corstens, Escher, & Romme, 2012; Romme, Escher, Dillon, Corstens, & Morris, 2009). What this really means is to better manage those parts of your social life from which these discourses are arising. Once again, you have to fix the bad situations in life, not try and fix the person.

14. *Dreams are another 'thinking' experience that can mix language responding, imagery, and other sensory responding.* Once again, the experience is very different, not because we have a totally new phenomenon, but because we are not engaging concurrently with the world at all during sleep. Unlike most imagery and thinking, what is experienced will consist of snippets of conversations, discourses, perceptual responding that have already occurred, albeit with no overarching organization like a 'me' thought stream, and contextualization of the real contexts is needed (Tedlock, 1987). This is what Freud, Jung, and others found, that the experiences of dreams was of chatter about the sleeper's main life problems and conflictual social situations, even for those thoughts that were almost never said out loud while awake (the really punished thoughts). They used dreams to help get the person to say out loud some of the thoughts that were punished when said out loud in real life.

15. *Prayer and talking to a god is another way people can refer to thinking experiences (for us, not for them).* For those who believe, the following is not aimed at them—they already can contextualize in their own way what is going on—and the thoughts obtained during prayer are external. The following is for those who do not believe, as an attempt to contextualize these forms of thinking so they will at least take such experiences as both real and important. However, not all forms of religion allow that God can speak directly to those in prayer, although most allow that you can get new thoughts and perspectives on your life when you pray.

The voices heard and the prayers (again, for non-believers) can be thought of as thoughts that are shaped outside of us in our many discursive communities, media, and social conversations (believers would say they are also shaped by an external spiritual presence), but that are not said out loud. Those praying or hearing god speak directly to them are not usually in bad situations like the 'voice hearers' usually are (see Chapter 3), but are part of a social group that let this experience occur, which is outside our normal experience of everyday thinking (Luhrmann, 2012). Hearing prayers and god speak directly, however, has long been reported to *first* occur when people are in bad situations (James, 1902/1958).

Prayer for the non-believers, therefore, can be framed as attending to all the many simultaneous language responses we are having that normally are not said out loud. Prayer gives us a chance to 'hear' these many thoughts never said out loud, just as Freud did with his methods. Indeed, there are many 'methods' of prayer within Christian religions and even more if one includes other religions and Buddhist practices. Some praying is very much about saying the 'me' voice thoughts, which often end up with prayers being direct pleas or requests to a god for help. Other forms stay more open so that repressed thoughts or thoughts that would be punished for being said out loud have more chance of being responded to. Such practices are common across many types of social experiences and vary greatly (Keating, 1992; LaDuke, 2005; Moore, 1992; Perry, 1999; Rouget, 1985; Ulanov & Ulanov, 1982; Zaleski & Zaleski, 2005). There have been periods in history during which similar practices were common without being attached to a religion at all (Hadot, 1995), similar to Buddhist practices.

The important point is that these thoughts/prayers will involve the person's everyday discourses in the worlds around them, and especially those that arise from bad or problematic situations, and so such practices can be very useful (if they are not just begging for favours from your god).

16. *Silence and isolation* have also been experiences in which voices or thoughts are recognized better and is a strong part of some religious traditions like Quakerism and Buddhism (Baumann, 1998; Birkel, 2004; Loring, 1992). Many people also speak of this as one positive feature of going deeply into nature, and especially when going alone. Silence and isolation have also historically been reported as leading to stronger experiences of our multiple thoughts and possibly becoming spiritual or religious afterwards (James, 1902/1958).

The point for us is that in silence or isolation there are no distractions from 'real' voices coming from other people or the dominance of the one language response that needs to be said next in conversational exchange (which normal therapy suffers from since you are engaged in conversation and cannot hear all your thoughts other than 'me' voices). Similar experiences are reported, of all the 'me' voices prattling on about immediate worries and concerns in the first instance (like the first 15 minutes of my first Quaker meeting experience), followed by other thoughts or voices or larger issues and thoughts, and then of thoughts that have been avoided or ignored for a long time but that are important to hear.

17. *Once there are contexts to hear the otherwise 'unconscious' thoughts, there is the question of what to do with them.* Freud had methods (Guerin, 2016) for working through these, and many traditions exists.

    There is a really interesting Quaker tradition of listening to 'voices' and working *with* those voices if they come from God. They call it 'discernment' (Fendall, Wood, & Bishop, 2007). For Quakers, in such a process one must first hear all the voices from sources that we cannot see (see the next section) and then discern which are from God and which are from your own 'ego' (what I have called in this book, the 'me' voice). Discernment leads to better decision-making and Quakers have procedures for doing this in groups, because they dislike or mistrust procedures of basic consensus.

    > We believe that God speaks with us all the time, whispering in our ears, nudging our emotions, stirring our senses, and drawing us to the preferred path. Even now, as you read these words, God may be stirring within you, calling, opening, and speaking to you. God desires to be your partner, to journey through life with you ... Both God and humans seek the reality of this dialogue and companionship. Spiritual discernment is the process of learning the language and the process of this relationship.
    >
    > (Fendall et al., 2007, p. 23)

    If you think back to V4.7, these are all useful ways to avoid the language 'gaps', which were a major problem arising from our overuse of language in our lives.

18. Since thinking comes from the discourses around us in our lives, it makes sense that *different experiences of thinking can occur when in strong social or community situations, not just when in salience or isolation.* I will give two examples. First, Quaker meetings usually consist of an hour of sitting in silence with a room full of people, no one talking. For me, this had a powerful effect and after some time lots of different thoughts 'pop into your head', which you might not ever have said but can recognize that they might have been present as unsaid language responses for a long time in your life. Second, many groups (almost all kin-based communities actually), have ceremonies with most of the community members present in which there is either talk or singing or both (DeNora, 2015; Gill, 1987; Graham, 1995; Guerin, 2020; Marett, 2005; Moyle, 1986; Seeger, 1987). These produce different 'thinking' experiences because the discursive audiences for everyday thinking are actually present! This means that community-important thinking (as

opposed to just the 'me voice') will appear and can become public depending on the specific practices.

Some of these have effects *and change the experiences of thinking* because they go on for a long time, and their repetition either distracts or gets rid of the 'me' voice thoughts (remember Titchener mentioned earlier). Some are over days (Moyle, 1986), while for the Suyá (Seeger, 1987), the men sang for 14 hours straight. These are examples of tight communities singing their community discourses that are not usually performed out loud, even if 'thought' sometimes by individuals. Over 14 hours the practice is not doing what Western therapies try to do and change or distract the 'individual' person's thoughts, but the practices *can directly reshape the entire discursive community's range of talk and thinking.* So, rather than a stranger therapist in an office trying to reshape your thinking discourses (see Chapter 5), these rituals reshape the ways the whole community talks in the first place, and new solutions to community issues will appear. *Direct social action instead of individual therapy!*

In another interesting example of directly changing the external discursive community, when the Xavante of Brazil have important community matters to discuss and make decisions from *all the thoughts spinning around the community* (not from inside their heads), the men get together at dusk and after an introduction they begin talking out loud simultaneously (Graham, 1995). They lie down, often in a circle with their heads towards the middle so they do not see each other, and often try to disguise their voice. Meanwhile it is dark, so like good Freudian clients, they are speaking out loud all of their thoughts (which are from the community discourses anyway, including unpopular ones and less preferred ideas, like Quaker discernment accomplishes). And everyone in the community can still hear them. This way, over a long period in the dark, all the possible community discourses and options are said out loud in front of everyone, both good and bad.

19. Following from the above, there have always been academics writings about so-called 'primitive' thinking and cultural differences in thinking. What seems clear is that *where the experience of thinking does seem different, this is not anything inherent in the people, but arises from the different forms of the discursive communities that shape the thoughts.* When thoughts are considered as arising from the social, cultural, and other discursive events in your world, the very experience of thinking would be expected to be different. People living in large family groups in a jungle did not get bombarded from birth by media and marketing shaping a range of diverse and useless discourses.

In point 18 above, we saw some examples of this happening. In V5.1 we saw that 'Western' discourses have progressively excluded any influence by social or community groups and have ended up with 'individualistic' notions of thinking rationally. I argued there that rationality really means 'non-social', since that has been excluded. So, any groups that have not been influenced by capitalism into assuming thinking is rational and is 'inside' them (we only seem to be 'individuals' because money allows that misconception), and that have their major external discourses arising from known kinship groups, will certainly experience 'thinking' differently—but having the discourse so close to the social community is certainly not 'primitive', just different. Their main thoughts will be about the community and its issues rather than what is individualistically the 'rational' thing to do for yourself in any situation. The 'me' voice will be more of an 'us' voice but not quite in the sense of Levy-Bruhl (1966) and others.

To put this another way, the so-called 'primitive mentalities' are really just 'community mentalities' and just as smart, savvy, and rational (Rasmussen, 2015). What we Westerners take to be standard thinking practices are shaped by our own social and cultural worlds just as much, but this means being shaped by capitalism, patriarchy, economics, bureaucracies, compartmentalization, individualism, social inequalities, etc., all features of the societies we live in and that shape us (V5 has more on this). In this sense, the Western forms of thinking experiences are the odd ones out on this planet!

20. There are many more anomalous experiences for humans that involve thinking experiences (Reed, 1974) but I cannot cover and contextualize them all. The main gist is to *treat thoughts as a case of language use shaped from our external discursive worlds, and then changing the thoughts or the social worlds will change that experience*. With 'fugue states' for example, I would begin to contextualize that the social shaping of thinking and talking in that person's life has become exclusively from generalized or societal audiences and no longer arises from real people. So, the thoughts no longer link to *specific* events going on. Interesting cases arise in hypnosis and how it socially affects thinking (Erickson, Rossi, & Rossi, 1976), and attention and absent mindedness, déjà vu, blurring of ego boundaries, thought broadcasting and thought insertion, and many more (Reed, 1974).

The main research question of this book

With that introduction to the peculiar aspects of analysing thinking, I can now set out the problem for this book. Acting, talking, and thinking are shaped by our many environments, which facilitate or constrain what we do. We are going in Chapter 4 to explore the possible ways in which the traditional 'behaviours of mental health' might be shaped by these environments even though these behaviours have been historically classed as 'mental' purely because their shaping environments are very difficult to see. A difficult task indeed.

What we will find is that a large number of these hidden shaping environments are based on social relationships, societal structures, and the use of language, and these have been overlooked. If you can sort these out, the bigger picture falls into place more easily. So, many of the problems are the same ones we have already discussed and include:

- The effects of social relationships (personal and societal) are difficult to observe.
- Language use is purely a social activity and more about the social dynamics than the words themselves that are said.
- It is difficult to see the effects of social relationships and discursive communities on language, especially when it is the form we call thinking (V4.4).
- Most of the spiritual effects are real and have been shaped by social and cultural contexts with very real material outcomes but that are difficult to observe.
- Most of the 'cognitive' phenomena have been shaped by social and cultural contexts and are really about language use (V4.8).
- A large proportion of the 'mental health' issues involve language and thinking issues.
- Societal structures shape our behaviours but are also difficult to see (economic systems, bureaucracies, patriarchy, colonization structures), and 'mental health' professionals are given no training in using a 'sociological imagination'.
- A key point that will be vital in Chapter 4 is that language, thinking, and imaging all originate in social relationships; so when there is a 'thinking disorder' or 'imaging disorder', you need to examine closely whether something is messed up in that person's social or societal relationships. Do not focus so much on the typography of the variations of the thinking but on why the person's relationships are not holding together a more 'normal' pattern of thinking.

Once we come to grips with better analyses of social and societal relationships and their effects, and how this plays out in using language, we will be in a better position to observe the environmental shapers of all the weird and wonderful things humans do, say, and think. Especially when they are in bad situations and cannot see where it is coming from.

References

Baumann, R. (1998). *Let your words be few: Symbolism of speaking and silence among seventeenth-century Quakers.* Cambridge, UK: Cambridge University Press.

Birkel, M. L. (2004). *Silence and witness: The Quaker tradition.* Maryknoll, NY: Orbis Books.

Deleuze, G. (1986). *Cinema 1: The movement-image.* Minneapolis: University of Minnesota Press.

Deleuze, G. (1989). *Cinema 2: The time image.* Minneapolis: University of Minnesota Press.

DeNora, T. (2015). *Music asylums: Wellbeing through music in everyday life.* London: Routledge.

Erickson, M. H., Rossi, E. L., & Rossi, S. I. (1976). *Hypnotic realities: The induction of clinical hypnosis and forms of indirect suggestion.* New York, NY: Irvington.

Fendall, L., Wood, J., & Bishop, B. (2007). *Practicing discernment together: Finding God's way forward in decision making.* Newberg, OR: Barclay Press.

Geyer, M. (2008). *Behind the wall: The women of the Destitute Asylum Adelaide, 1852–1918.* Adelaide: Wakefield Press.

Gibson, J. J. (1971). On the relation between hallucination and perception. *Leonardo, 3,* 425–427.

Gibson, J. J. (1978). The ecological approach to the visual perception of picture. *Leonardo, 11,* 227–235.

Gibson, J. J. (1979). *An ecological approach to visual perception.* Boston, MA: Houghton Mifflin.

Gill, S. (1987). *Native American religious action: A performative approach to religion.* Columbia: University of South Carolina Press.

Graham, L. R. (1995). *Performing dreams: Discourses of immortality among the Xavante of Central Brazil.* Austin: University of Texas Press.

Guerin, B. (1990). Gibson, Skinner, and perceptual responses. *Behavior and Philosophy, 18,* 43–54.

Guerin, B. (2016). *How to rethink human behavior: A practical guide to social contextual analysis.* London: Routledge.

Guerin, B. (2017). *How to rethink mental illness: The human contexts behind the labels.* London: Routledge.

Guerin, B. (2018). The use of participatory and non-experimental research methods in behavior analysis. *Revista Perspectivas em Anályse Comportamento, 9,* 248–264.

Guerin, B. (2019a). Contextualizing music to enhance music therapy. *Revista Perspectivas em Anályse Comportamento, 10,* 222–242.

Guerin, B. (2019b). What do therapists and clients talk about when they cannot explain behaviours? How Carl Jung avoided analysing a client's environments by inventing theories. *Revista Perspectivas em Anályse Comportamento, 10,* 76–97.

Guerin, B., Leugi, G. B., & Thain, A. (2018). Attempting to overcome problems shared by both qualitative and quantitative methodologies: Two hybrid procedures to encourage diverse research. *Australian Community Psychologist, 29*, 74–90.

Hadot, P. (1995). *Philosophy as a way of life: Spiritual exercises from Socrates to Foucault*. London: Blackwell.

James, W. (1902/1958). *The varieties of religious experience: A study in human nature*. New York, NY: New American Library.

Johnstone, L., Boyle, M., Cromby, J., Dillon, J., Harper, D., Kinderman, P., ... Read, J. (2018). *The Power Threat Meaning Framework: Towards the identification of patterns in emotional distress, unusual experiences and troubled or troubling behaviour, as an alternative to functional psychiatric diagnosis*. Leicester, UK: British Psychological Society.

Keating, T. (1992). *Open mind, open heart: The contemplative dimension of the Gospel*. Shaftesbury, UK: Element.

Kinderman, P. (2019). *A manifesto for mental health: Why we need a revolution in mental health care*. London: Palgrave Macmillan.

LaDuke, W. (2005). *Recovering the sacred: The power of naming and claiming*. Chicago, IL: Haymarket Books.

Levy-Bruhl, L. (1966). *The 'soul' of the primitive*. Chicago, IL: Henry Regnery.

Longden, E., Corstens, D., Escher, S., & Romme, M. (2012). Voice hearing in a biographical context: A model for formulating the relationship between voices and life history. *Psychosis, 4*, 224–234.

Loring, P. (1992). *Spiritual discernment: The context and goal of clearness committees*. Wallingford, PA: Pendle Hill Publications.

Luhrmann, T. M. (2012). *When God talks back: Understanding the American evangelical relationships with God*. New York, NY: Vintage Books.

Marett, A. (2005). *Songs, dreamings, and ghosts: The Wangga of North Australia*. Middletown, CO: Wesleyan University press.

Moore, T. (1992). *Care of the soul: A guide for cultivating depth and sacredness in everyday life*. New York, NY: Harper Perennial.

Moyle, R. M. (1986). *Alyawarra music: Songs and society in a central Australian community*. Canberra: Australian Institute of Aboriginal Studies.

Perry, T. W. (1999). *Trials of the visionary mind: Spiritual emergency and the renewal process*. New York: State University of New York Press.

Rasmussen, S. (2015). An ambiguous spirit dream and Tuareg-Kunta relationships in rural Northern Mali. *Anthropological Quarterly, 88*, 635–664.

Reed, G. (1974). *The psychology of anomalous experience: A cognitive approach*: Boston, MA: Houghton Mifflin.

Romme, M., Escher, S., Dillon, J., Corstens, D., & Morris, M. (2009). *Living with voices: 50 stories of recovery*. London: PCCS Books.

Rouget, G. (1985). *Music and trance: A theory of the relations between music and possession*. Chicago, IL: University of Chicago Press.

Rose, A. M. (1962). A social-psychological theory of neurosis. In A. M. Rose (Ed.), *Human behavior and social processes: An interactionist approach* (pp. 537–549). Boston, MA: Houghton Mifflin.

Ryle, G. (1971). The thinking of thoughts: What is 'Le Penseur' doing? In G. Ryle, *Collected papers. Volume 2, collected essays 1929–1968* (pp. 480–496). London: Hutchinson.

Scalabrini, A., Mucci, C., Esposito, R., Damiani, S., & Northoff, G, (2020). Dissociation as a disorder of integration: On the footsteps of Pierre Janet. *Progress in Neuropsychopharmacology & Biological Psychiatry*, 101, 1–12.

Seeger, A. (1987). *Why Suyá sing: A musical anthropology of an Amazonian people.* Cambridge, UK: Cambridge University Press.

Tedlock, B. (Ed.) (1987). *Dreaming: Anthropological and psychological interpretations.* Santa Fe, NM: School of American Research Press.

Ulanov, A., & Ulanov, B. (1982). *Primary speech: A psychology of prayer.* Louisville, KY: Westminster John Knox Press.

Watson, J. (2019). *Drop the disorder: Challenging the culture of psychiatric diagnosis.* London: PCCS Books.

Woodiwiss, J. C. (1950). *Mad or bad? Studies of criminal insanity or wilful wrongdoing.* London: Quality Press.

Zaleski, P., & Zaleski, C. (2005). *Prayer: A history.* New York, NY: Houghton Mifflin.

3   What are the bad situations that lead to the 'mental health' behaviours and other outcomes?

There are bad situations in life that you can be born into or happen to find yourself in. People try and escape such conditions or at least evade the consequences, often getting into worse bad situations (cf. Maté, 2009). Most bad situations we manage to change or escape easily; this happens regularly in life but we either have support or resources to do something about these bad situations. Where things are worse, chronic, or we have no resources or skills (history) to change the bad situation, there are a myriad of ways people are then shaped to avoid, escape from, or change their bad life situations; some of these 'solutions' hurt other people and lead to more problems, and some involve just putting up with the suffering (even over a whole lifetime, sadly). But other bad situations get to a point in which unusual behaviours are shaped because all else has failed; these are normal behaviours, but they have been pushed to the extreme and become exaggerated. And some, but only some, get labelled 'mental health' when they match the (artificial) criteria in Chapter 2. Here are some examples of living with bad situations:

- Many times, bad situations just require *a few adjustments to life* and things gradually get better (e.g. a close friend passes away very suddenly and this is despairing, but you take a few days off work, get social support with family and friends, and eventually you find a way to cope with and move on from this bad situation).
- Sometimes people are getting some of their resource–social relationship pathways met even when in a bad situation, so *they put up with the bad parts* of their contexts (although the effects of this going on for years can end up being a bigger bad situation). This will not be viewed as a 'mental health' problem until it gets worse. For example, in the middle of last century it was expected that women would get married and have children (patriarchy) and many women did this even though they might rather have done something else with their life.

- Sometimes the 'bad part' of people's life is obvious and so *they know what to try and change*, and they can work with lawyers, police, social workers, and others to help with this (they are poor and try to budget better, and put up with the bad poverty situation and its many consequences in the meanwhile, hoping things will clear up).
- Through all of the attempts to deal with bad life situations, people are also remarkable in how they can *distract themselves* from their bad situations and suffering, to an extent (e.g. with entertainment, drugs, cultural practices, talking strategies, repetitive life practices).
- Sometimes there is a very bad situation (a 'traumatic event') that might only be of short duration but can change all the other contexts of the person's life. For example, even with car accidents or rape, these bad events can reshape (or even stop) a person's normal social relationships. They find it difficult to talk even to their family and friends, and this can then also change their economic opportunities, which changes their resource base, and all of which change how they present themselves (V5.6). So that in turn changes all their social relationships from what they had been prior to the traumatic event; so their life is now full of bad situations even though the event itself is long gone (V2.6).
- Sometimes the 'bad part' of a person's life is obvious and *they know what to try and change, but these solutions do not fit into their society's 'normal patterns'* of behaviours, so they end up doing legal but alternative activities such as communal or nomadic living of different forms to avoid the societal codes; music, and the other arts; living rough; rebelling against the society's 'normal patterns' of behaviours in roles of agitation and societal change; or living a 'bohemian lifestyle' as a 'disaffected youth', which has always existed in modernity even though it has gone by different names. This group might not be overly violent or risk-taking, but neither do they act 'normal' and just put up with not being happy as society expects—they explore alternative ways of behaving and living life *without engaging with the mainstream of society* (Cohen, 1971; Cohen & Taylor, 1976; Eckert, 1989; Glasper, 2006; Nordhoff, 1875/1966; Orwell, 1933; Rowe, 2018; Sartwell, 2014). These strategies also heavily depend upon societal stratification, so they break into groups based on race, class, wealth, etc. as to what is possible (a person in poverty 'dropping out' is very different from a person of wealth 'dropping out').
- Sometimes things are very bad with few alternative life strategies possible and most 'normal' ways to escape the bad situation are not viable or blocked, and so people *try some non-normal behaviours*, including illegal activities (Decker & van Winkle, 1996; Truong, 2018; Yablonsky, 1962), to change things and escape the bad situations

(e.g. using bullying, violence, strong interpersonal control, lying and deceiving, exploiting others, or crime).

- But sometimes people do not really know they are in a bad situation (their own contextual observations and discourses do not show that things are going wrong, but nothing seems to ever go well or according to their plans) and *they develop actions, talking, or thinking that mess with their life or with people in their life* but that *might just* change things (they might cry a lot at unexpected times but their observations and discourses have no awareness of the bad situations shaping this; the behaviours just seem to happen); so these behaviours appear to come out of nowhere and can get labelled as 'mental health' issues.

- Sometimes people know they are in a bad situation but with few alternative strategies possible and most 'normal' ways to escape the bad situation are not viable or are blocked, and *they have little choice but to just continue* even though they do not want to just put up with it and are not getting any resource–social relationship pathways; and *they then develop actions, talking, or thinking that mess with their life or with the people in their life* (but that might just change things); these also appear to come from nowhere and can get labelled as 'mental health' issues.

Remember through this that people switch between these depending on changes in their life contexts, and they can belong to more than one (called 'comorbid' when the 'mental health' labels are applied). For example, with 'disaffected youth' there are many varieties ranging from 'peaceful' hippies to sometimes violent skinheads. The point is that they are all in bad situations and being shaped to find solutions depending upon what is possible and available.

'Mental health' behaviours are only one possible outcome of these different strategies for dealing with bad situations, and we should stop making a strict distinction between all these because such distinctions are artificial. And as we saw in the last chapter, the label of 'mental health' is arbitrary because it always depends on how hard you have looked for the bad situations that are shaping the behaviours. The bad situations and the suffering are painful and are not arbitrary, but calling them 'mental health' is arbitrary.

Following Chapter 2, the last two points in the previous list are the ones that will typically be labelled 'mental health' issues, even though they only differ by degrees, by available resources and attempted social strategies, from the rest. Whether or not solutions to life's problems are possible depend on the world the person happens to be in: the resources they happen to have, their life experiences and history, their family and friendship networks, etc. Those raised in a world of using bullying and violence to get what you need are likely to try that strategy when they happen to be in a bad situation, and that might work (for them) even if they do not 'like' doing that. They might get referred to police and social workers at some point in their life but maybe not 'mental health' services.

The role of bad situations in producing 'mental health' issues and other behaviours

The basic idea is that *in bad situations and conflict situations people find ways to adapt or escape, using whatever they can and whatever they have available.* This all depends upon how severe the bad situation is, how it has already affected them, which alternatives actions are blocked, and what they are still getting back while living in such situations. But this also means that *we can look at all these cases together and focus our attention on how to understand and stop the bad situations* (Pathway 2), rather than attributing what happens to bad things inside a person and trying to change things 'inside' the person (Pathway 1). *We need to try and fix people's bad situations rather than trying to fix the person,* and 'mental health' outcomes are only some of the outcomes of living in bad situations.

People in bad situations can try as many solutions as they can, but this depends on their history and what is available in their context, which can change. If you are in poverty you cannot buy solutions, although thinking about stealing money or winning the lottery might be frequent. Notice that these solutions can vary and change; a person might try one that does not work and then try another. But how a person tries to solve or escape their bad life situations depends upon the situation or context, not some 'inner willpower'.

We will see in the next chapter that many topographically similar 'mental health' behaviours occur across many bad situations, not because they are 'hard-wired' but because they are the only alternatives left to try to change the bad situations—all others have been blocked. In the absence of anything else, people can always still cry, be violent, self-harm or complain of bodily pains, withdraw from all social contact, mess with their food patterns, etc. These behaviours are not 'hard-wired' but are sometimes the only remaining behaviours available that might be able to change their lot in life.

Our conclusion, then, is that we must change our focus to try and fix the bad situations (whether 'mental health' issues or bullying behaviour) instead of trying to change the person!

Let me repeat a bit by spelling out more details for four of the cases given above, although this is not meant as an analysis. All four can occur for people simultaneously for different parts of their lives, for example. What follows are four conceptual examples of situations that go from just normal conflicts to what might be considered bad situations. What I am trying to do here is shape you to stop looking 'inside' the people for the problems and solutions (Pathway 1), which was only ever a metaphor, and to look more closely into the people's life contexts for the problems and available solutions (Pathway 2). I will add here that finding and understanding the bad situations that have shaped the behaviours, does not legally condone those solutions. There is a strict distinction in Western life that understanding why a person did a crime does not excuse them from responsibility. If I was raised in bad circumstances and started criminal activities, I cannot be excused legally from a later crime because of that, in Western law. We can understand how it all developed but in a Western law court you will still be charged, although your sentence might be reduced in consideration of your bad circumstances.

Think of examples from your own life or experience of others and consider the following:

1. *There can be 'normal' bad situations that are limited, or that we can find solutions to with some easier social strategies.* For example, we might talk to friends and try and change our social relationships, find distractions from the worse parts or avoid them with entertainment, or put up with the situation because there is other good coming from the broader way of life. If you have capital or other resources you might be able to buy your way out through new solutions, you could also try to talk your way out of a situation if you have the resources to back up your talk, or if you have ways to control those around you. If you have no one to talk to about the problem (but have money) you could try psychotherapy or go to other professionals such as law courts, the police, counsellors, mediation services, financial advisors, self-improvement courses, 'life coaches', etc.

   It is also very common that people are just not happy with their life circumstances, but cannot do much about this because of constraints, lack of experience, lack of opportunities, or lack of resources. They *put up with* the circumstances (perhaps with social discourses about escaping in the future), and they distract themselves from the problems through drugs and entertainment of all sorts, limiting their discourses around future expectations, and distractions of all sorts that give them some good outcomes in the short term.

2. *If there are bad situations with no obvious or 'normal' solutions possible but the problems in the environments are salient or obvious, then more extreme solutions will be shaped.* These can include ubiquitous violence, bullying, lying and deceiving, and crime. These can also include more extreme solutions that change the environment more drastically, such as excluding people from your life or moving away

physically from situations, but mostly avoidance or escape strategies
because the bad situation itself is known but not easily solved.

3. *There can be bad situations with no obvious or easy origin to be seen
   nor solutions to be found.* The conflicts and 'badness' are arising from
   the person's environments or contexts but it is not obvious where they
   are coming from ("Nothing ever works out for me and I don't know
   why"; "I should be grateful I know, but I am just not happy with things
   and I don't know why"; "Why do the men at work always get opportunities given to them but not us women?").

   In such situations the responses can be varied but move between violence and bullying to get out or change things, attempting the 'normal'
   strategies such as talking your way out (but who do you talk to when the
   sources are hidden?), and *exaggerating* 'normal' strategies when they
   do not work (if you are running out of options). Part of the problem
   here is that most bad situations are bad because the person has already
   been limited in what they are able to do and change in their life, so
   already many possible options and 'normal' strategies for changing
   your world are not available. For example, in many bad and oppressive
   situations people are silenced so no language strategies will be possible, despite language-use strategies probably being the most common
   way we change our normal life situations (V4.3).

4. *There are very bad situations in which other options are blocked, you
   cannot observe where the problems are coming from, and all attempts at
   change do not work out.* Here, people are shaped by their contexts (they
   do not choose this verbally) into doing almost 'any other behaviours'
   they can to change things and to then exaggerate these behaviours if
   they do not work. This is where, it is argued, some of the more unusual
   or extreme 'mental health' behaviours arise.

   For example, if behaviour has been controlled and limited by the
   people or society (e.g. patriarchy) in a situation, so there are few
   behaviours left available to change it, then what will be shaped in these
   circumstances? Even in such situations, disruptions to food and eating
   practices can be shaped since they will always exist, withdrawal from
   all activities and social relationships can be shaped, exaggerated talking
   out loud can be shaped since this has historically been what produces
   change in other people's behaviour, and exaggerated talking but not
   out loud (i.e. thinking) can be shaped until people hear the wildest and
   most anxious thoughts and 'voices'.

So, it is suggested that the cauldron of all these possible social actions
within bad situations shape most 'mental health' behaviours, but I argue that
the distinction between 'mental health' behaviours and 'non-mental health'

behaviours is nebulous. If there was a simpler solution then people would have done it and the behaviour would not be classified as a 'mental health' issue. If the situation was bad but they resorted to bullying, crime or violence, then it would also not even be classified as a 'mental health' issue *per se.* This is why the Power Threat Meaning Framework (PTMF) 'change of question' is important: do not ask someone in such circumstances "What is wrong with you?" but instead ask, "What has happened to you?" (Johnstone et al., 2018). I am just expanding this beyond what are called 'mental health' behaviours.

Three guides to help see bad situations as the contexts shaping many difficult behaviours

The following are three guides to help your transition from asking "What is wrong with you?" to asking, "What has happened to you?" To transition from Pathway 1 to Pathway 2. They are guides to shape you to examine the person's contexts more closely and not make internal attributions (Guerin, 2016).

Guide 1: some observable contexts of bad situations and different 'solutions'

Table 3.1 gives some examples of observable conditions, but which of those end up getting labelled 'mental health' issues is not a clear distinction, and only loosely based on (1) how many alternatives solutions have been blocked, and (2) whether the bad conditions can be observed easily or not. The point is that *we need to focus on changing the bad situations* and this includes many bad life situations that have been hitherto artificially separated from those labelled as 'mental health' issues.

Guide 2: some general life conflict situations that can become bad situations

The examples in Box 3.1 are more abstract but might help you to think about some of the general life conflict situations from which bad situations can arise, regardless of whether they get called 'mental health' issues or not. Notice that because these are in terms of resource–social relationship pathways *they are not about individuals* but *about individuals within social and societal systems*—people in their environments (Guerin, 2016, V5.3). For example, 'lack of skills to obtain resources' can be due to the socio-economic situation in which the person was born rather than anything about their capabilities as a human being; given a new environment, they might become very capable (Haley, 1973). Furthermore, 'competing relationships' are currently heavily shaped as a result of what we learn from being socialized within our capitalist economic system, it is not meant as a personal 'trait'.

Table 3.1 Descriptions of different bad situations in life and the various behaviours that can be shaped

Different ways of thinking about the various bad situations in life

The least → The worst
'Normal' social conflicts and resource limitations → Most alternative behaviours not possible or blocked
Easy to analyse conflicts and to find solutions → Difficult to analyse conflicts and no easy solutions available
Not labelled as 'mental health' issue → Gets labelled as 'mental health' issue

'Normal' bad situations that we can analyse more or less easily and we can find solutions with some social support and strategies	Bad situations that we can analyse more or less easily but need others to help us solve (e.g. lawyers, police, social workers)	Bad situations that we can analyse more or less easily but the 'normal solutions' require being more 'normal' and so the person disengages from the mainstream to deal with this; they do not fit into their society's 'normal patterns' of behaviours, which in turn removes some solutions	Bad situations that we can analyse more or less easily but the problems in the environment would require more extreme solutions, so people just put up with it	Bad situations that we can analyse more or less easily but the problems in the environment require more extreme solutions, which can include violence, lying and deceiving, bullying, and crime	Bad situations that are difficult to analyse, with no obvious or easy origin to be seen nor solutions to be found. The conflicts and badness arising from the person's contexts are not salient and they have little choice but to just continue. If they cannot do any of the above available behaviours will become extreme and affect resources and social relationships	Very bad situations in which other options are blocked, you cannot observe where the problems are even coming from, and all attempts at change do not work out. Here, people are shaped into almost 'any other behaviours' they can do, to change things. They develop actions, talking, or thinking that mess with their life or with people in their life but that *might* just change things

---

Box 3.1 Some ways in which bad life situations arise when considered through resource–social relationship pathways

Too much stress and conflict in obtaining life resources (resources in a broad sense)

Getting resources is blocked due to lack of opportunities or lack of social relationships, either through limited opportunities, lacking the life skills needed, or lacking the extensive stories to obtain relationships and resources.

Too much stress in life social relationships

Social conflicts in relationships, competing relationships, pressure of image management for social relationships, lacking the social skills needed, serious language confusions from audience pressures, needs extensive stories to manage competing relationships.

Conflicting ways of obtaining resources

Competing sources, competing opportunities, lacking the skills needed, needs extensive stories to mitigate conflict.

Conflicting audiences and social relationships

Producing strongly conflicting thoughts and thinking patterns from negotiating, conflicting audiences brought together somehow, lacking the skills needed, serious language confusions arising from conflicting audiences, needs extensive stories to mitigate conflict.

Strategies out of control or locked in

Bluff games gone wrong, bluff games using relationships (includes double binds), competition gone wrong, social traps escalating badly, lacking the skills needed, multiple thoughts produced from strategies that might be conflicting or confusing, needs extensive stories to make strategies work.

These two guides alone do not tell us much, but the aim is to help put life conflicts for people into an external contextual framework rather than 'inside' the head of the individuals. Each of these conflict situations, of course, are set within societal contexts that create and maintain the conflicts. These have been outlined more fully in V5.3 and Guerin (2016).

Bad situations can therefore arise from all sorts of problems with resource–social relationship pathways. They can range from mild disagreements with your friends and family to major traumatic incidents that tear your life apart (i.e. negatively affect *all* your contexts). Some are easily fixed by changing your environments (social, economic, etc.) and others are not (poverty, patriarchy, capitalism).

Bad situations shape many responses, which include, but are not limited to, 'mental health' issues. Severe childhood adversity can shape not only 'mental health' issues (Johnstone et al., 2018) but also violence, bullying, withdrawal from 'normal' life patterns that are not categorized as 'mental health' problems, or else have a very blurred boundary. We should not be studying, analysing, and working with 'mental health' behaviours as if they were categorially separate. We should be working with *all behaviours shaped by bad situations in life*, and those currently singled out as relevant to 'mental health' or 'psychological health' issues are just those occurring when the bad situations cannot be observed easily and the people have few or no alternative responses available and are trapped.

Guide 3: the contexts of bad situations and their severity or pain

Here is another way to guide you to look at the person's context rather than 'inside' their head. There is a misconception, I believe, in how *severity* is linked to those behaviours singled out as 'mental health'. As we saw in the last chapter (see also Guerin, 2017), whether something is called a 'psychological' or 'mental health' issue is a judgement made by professionals, and the basis for it is not necessarily related to the severity. Rather, if the person's situations are bad but *cannot be seen easily*, even if they seem mild, then this gets attributed to a 'psychological' or a 'mental' problem. And as we saw, there are many reasons why the bad contexts might not be noticed, and these have nothing to do with the severity of pain or suffering.

This also flows through the history of therapy (at least how I presented it, in Chapter 1). It was *the difficulty in seeing where the new problem behaviours came from* that shaped Janet, Freud, and others into their abstract discourses about 'psychological' or 'unconscious' problems when no neurological basis was found. I argued instead that many of these behaviours really stemmed from changes in societal systems, which were not easily seen.

So, the pain or severity is not directly related to whether a situation seems bad to a professional or to the person in the situation. The severity depends on whether a situation can be observed to be bad or not *once they are properly contextualized*. The worst life situations are not always those called 'mental health'. People have very bad life situations for which they can see the problem situation but cannot not do much about it and just put up with it (they are likely to drift in and out of 'mental health' issues). When talking about the 'mental health' (or not) bad life situations, we are always talking about the *observability* of the situations, not necessarily the *severity*. We need to attend to all the behaviours arising from bad situations in life. This is why developing a 'sociological imagination' (Mills, 1959) is vital to all professionals, because these are commonly the bad situations not easily seen.

This has all been a source of confusion since the beginning of the twentieth century until now (hopefully). The difference between 'normal' behaviours (even violence and crime) and 'mental health' behaviours has seemed like a categorical difference. The 'mental health' behaviours, while resembling everyday behaviours, have seemed like something different that people are doing—they involve the 'mind' or a brain disease. However, the difference is in the *bad situations and their observabilities*, not in the behaviours themselves or their observabilities.

The behaviours themselves are 'normal' behaviours reshaped into problems (see Chapter 4). Normal behaviours do not by themselves become critical 'mental health' issues. It is the bad situations in life that become painful quagmires in which 'mental health' behaviours are shaped from those everyday behaviours, but these quagmires also shape a lot of other behaviours, which never get called 'mental health' problems. *We all need to work together to fix the bad situations rather than trying to fix the person.*

What are the bad situations?

The everyday conflicts around resources and social relationships can become entrenched in various ways, within which finding alternatives or escapes are both blocked and the person gets trapped. Some arise within everyday conflicts while others are a result of the way society as a whole limits what people can and cannot do, although almost every conflict partly arises because of the structuring of societal opportunities for resources and for social relationships.

Contexts for bad situations

Common bad situations are those that involve:

- violence;
- crime;
- drugs used as common 'solutions', perhaps distraction at first;

- poverty;
- traumatic events of all sorts, long term or short term (like car accidents);
- abuse of all sorts (physical, sexual, power, control, etc.);
- combat and fighting, both for those fighting and those escaping the combat situations;
- oppression and violent control taken by individuals or groups;
- bullying over time, especially at school, work, in the family;
- lack of opportunities for other reasons, or silencing;
- strong restrictions imposed on many behaviours that become blocked;
- exclusion or discrimination from social relationships (and hence resources and support);
- having disabilities and less flexible behaviour repertoires that restrict opportunities, including major illnesses;
- feeling that you just do not 'fit in' to the world you were born into (hard to generalize what contexts shape this, however);
- hospitalization itself, especially when enforced, and the use of medically prescribed drugs that change a lot of irrelevant behaviours also with unwanted effects (cf. Dembo & Hanfmann, 1935).

Points to note

- All the above are treated as contexts in which a person finds themselves, and most are situations people find themselves in through no fault of their own. Indeed, many are situations into which people have been born.
- Poverty does not necessarily mean 'trauma' in the usual sense, but is a bad situation because it prevents so many opportunities in the current capitalist world. So people living in poverty contexts can find themselves in other bad situations and might not be able to change their situations easily with few resources.
- People can appear to be in good situations and be happy but are not. Wealthy people can be in bad situations despite their background, but the difference is that they can usually find ways of 'buying themselves' out of such situations and opening up other opportunities that are blocked for most. Wealth does not prevent 'mental health' so much as allow for more solutions in order to change any bad situations which arise.
- Children are especially vulnerable because of the following:
    - They have limited repertoires of behaviours to escape and rely on only a few that are easily available (e.g. withdrawal, self-harm, food disruptions, social relationship disruptions).

- They have little access to resources or capital to buy the solutions through other people in the way that adults might.
- They have fewer language strategies available to talk their way out of things and few resources anyway to reciprocate in order to make the language work and change people.
- They are more likely to be persuaded by local adults that the situation is 'normal' and there is nothing needing changing.
- Bullying in schools shows these problems when compared to adult bullying. Some children in such bad situations are often found to have been shaped into more adult social strategies out of necessity in their attempts to cope.
- Some bad situations include a large number of these problems. Colonization and slavery produced most of the bad situations listed above simultaneously, for both those immediately affected and for their descendants (e.g. Wyatt-Brown, 1988; see Chapter 8). Minority groups in any society also tend to be in multiple bad situations (Qi, Palmier-Claus, Simpson, Varese, & Bentall, 2019; Riggs & Treharne, 2017).

The cases of 'trauma' and more blurry distinctions

Some people have experienced bad traumatic events and yet still cope and continue their everyday life, but this depends on their resource–social relationship pathways and the opportunities to maintain these. If a traumatic event severely compromises *most* of their *other* life contexts (V2.6), then this will badly affect their future resource–social relationship pathways and continue their suffering even if the event itself was short-lived. Experiencing a traumatic event most often is likely to affect social relationship contexts. For example, the person might withdraw from normal conversations to avoid being put on the spot about their traumatic experiences and this will often dramatically change their life for the worse. Or they might have the capital to deal with their bad situation and suffering after a traumatic experience, so few contexts are changed very much.

So, the point is to not focus solely on the original bad or traumatic event but rather to *explore how that event changed all the other life contexts subsequently* and affected any resource–social relationship pathways the person had at the time (cf. Bovin & Marx, 2011; Guerin, 2017), and thereby left them in an even bigger bad situation. There are cases where people are able to cope with the original traumatic event and seem fine afterwards, but the subsequent ways in which this changes that person's other contexts gradually becomes a bad situation in itself later on. For example, a family might cope well in many ways with the death of a parent, but the subsequent

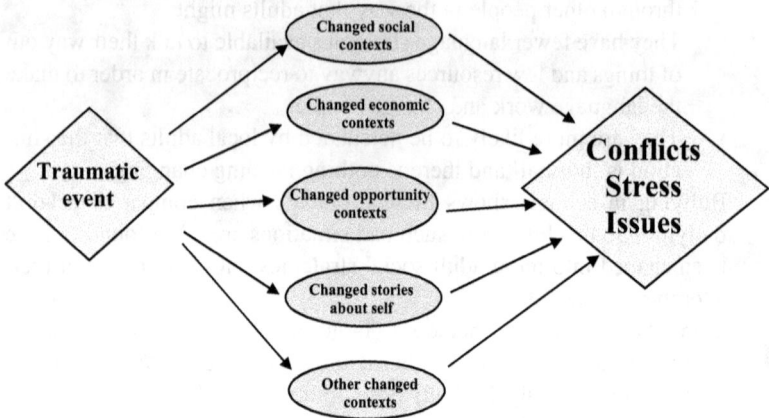

Figure 3.1 How current issues might have arisen from the ways in which early
traumatic events or bad life situations changed many contexts at the
time rather than those events themselves

changes in both economic and social relationship contexts because of this
event might present a persistent bad situation that is less easy to deal with
later on (see Figure 3.1).

In other cases of bad situations, however, there are no actual 'traumatic
events' but the person's lack of opportunities through birth or subsequent
events means they have been trapped in a bad situation over a long time with
few alternatives or ways out, and this is just as devastating. So, situations
that are typically labelled as 'traumatic' are usually bad, but they are not the
only bad situations.

Finally, some people can survive and even thrive through these bad situations, but we should never take this for granted. This is not because they
have magical internal properties of 'resilience' or 'willpower', but because
of other parts of their external contexts that were in place. We need to study
these contextually and find out more (Hartman, 2019).

Ways that the 'solutions' shaped by bad situations can affect a person's contexts

So, the upshot is that early traumatic events are important and bad, but we
also need to find out how people's contexts were *changed* by those traumatic events and subsequently shaped their lives in other directions. Notice
again that I am trying to shape readers to focus on the person's life situations (Pathway 2) and not some 'inner worlds' (Pathway 2). Table 3.2 is
a guide to sensitize readers to 'see' all these contexts when they work with

Table 3.2 Some bad situations in life and common life contexts that might have been collaterally affected in adverse ways

Bad situations	Possible effects on other contexts in that person's worlds
Violence	Increases secrecy, therefore, increases thinking over talking Trains people further in the use of violence and bullying as solutions Becomes locked in as further violence is usually a consequence Trains for escape and avoidance strategies in life Difficulties with bureaucracies and 'societal controls' as violence is not tolerated as a social strategy
Crime	Increases secrecy, therefore increases thinking over talking Becomes locked in Trains for escape and avoidance strategies in life
Drugs	Can prevent trying other solutions to bad situations Become a solution to *any* bad situation Becomes locked in In some cases, economic resources are needed that causes other issues Need for secrecy if illegal or taken to excess, so some social relationships become altered and some supportive people lost
Poverty	Difficulty getting resources Difficulty getting social relationships of all sorts since that requires money in modernity Difficult to find other solutions for bad situations with no money In modern society lack of money restricts almost all access and opportunities for resources In modern society lack of money restricts almost all access and opportunities for social relationship building Restricts the 'power' of discourses to have any effect within social relationships
Short-term traumatic events (e.g. rape, car accident)	Needs new stories and self-narratives to portray world Avoid social relationships if difficult to talk about Often physical damage so new medical contexts to deal with that can also alter previous social relationships Sometimes economic contexts are changed and so resources are changed
Long-term traumatic events or abuse (e.g. physical, sexual, power, control)	Increases secrecy, therefore increases thinking over talking 'Dissociated' stories and self-narratives gradually used to portray world Social relationships become contradictory and compartmentalized Thinking and talk become contradictory and compartmentalized

(*continued*)

Table 3.2 Cont.

Bad situations	Possible effects on other contexts in that person's worlds
	Avoidance of social relationships to avoid stories
	Long-term means more difficult to change, becomes locked in
	Controlling social relationships will change most other life contexts
Oppression and violent control taken by individuals or groups	Social relationships become contradictory and compartmentalized
	Controlling social relationships will change most other life contexts
	'Disassociated' stories and self-narratives gradually used to portray world if able to talk to people outside the controlling relationship
Lack of opportunities	Whether through poverty, oppressive control, or disabilities, most other life contexts are changed
Exclusion or discrimination from social relationships	Resources coming through those relationships are now impossible
Having disabilities and less flexible behaviour repertoires	Restricts opportunities
	Restricts social relationships
	Many contextual restrictions that can probably be avoided but need social support

someone. Every person will be different, but this might help sensitize you to begin asking the right questions.

Societal contexts for bad situations

With the large populations in modern Western societies, and the increasing replacement of family social relationships with stranger or contractual social relationships, the way society as a whole is structured and how this structuring is enforced through strangers (bureaucracies, police) now produces many *new* bad situations for people (see Chapter 1).

Previous subsistence-style kin-based groups had other sorts of bad situations, but they were mostly resolved because the source of the problems was known. The main big dilemma was in the *vicissitudes of nature*, when bad situations in the community arose from drought, diseases, and other 'natural' disasters. A lot of 'non-everyday social behaviours' were shaped as a result of these.

Box 3.2 includes some brief notes on common society-produced bad situations from which many people suffer through no fault of their own (the focus is on current modern Western societies). More is summarized elsewhere on the shaping of these (see Guerin, 2004, 2016, 2019, V5.3).

Box 3.2 Some ways in which societal 'structures' can directly shape people's behaviours

Societal effects on social relationships (includes language use; V4.3)

- Issues arising within families and how they are now negatively affected by stranger relationships and the effects of capitalism.
- Issues arising from social properties of strangers especially having to negotiate resource–social relationship pathways with strangers.
- Issues arising from requiring more strangers to deal with stranger problems.
- The effects from having little choice of or influence over stranger relationships.
- Violence strategies used within social relationships when family options for control have been blocked by capitalism.
- A lack of language to get people to do things other than through monetary reciprocity.

Economics effects in a broad sense (how we get things in order to live)

- Our resources and resource distribution are very constrained by the capitalist system, we cannot change these easily, and we are all constrained by resource opportunities and barriers that existed before we were born.
- It is very difficult or impossible to escape the effects of capitalism.
- Capitalism produces poverty and inequalities as part of the way it works, so many people will be trapped inside poverty.
- As mentioned earlier, poverty is a bad situation because most ways of changing the situation or changing people within the situations now require money to work.

Patriarchy

- Bad situations arise from the systemic societal constraints on how males and females are shaped to behave differently, mostly to restrict female opportunities.
- There are large historic inequalities between genders for both resources and resource distribution, and the behaviours within social relationships and what is allowed.
- These inequalities are far-reaching in people's lives still although enacted by strangers now.

Cultural practices

- Within our cultural groups (whether family, community, or strangers) there are constraints on how we need to behave in order to keep access to group resources.
- Being part of a cultural group can entail ostracism if it does not conform to cultural practices, although such cultural groups can also be the most supportive in times of conflict, meaning that people often remain and 'put up' with some issues.

Colonization

- Colonization produced almost all the other bad situations for those who were colonized, usually simultaneously (see Chapter 7 for more).

Societal oppressions

- Control by modern societal authorities trying to deal with huge populations, capitalism, and bureaucracies leads to many new bad situations.
- These new bad situations include societal uses of economic controls, the use of societal force through police and the military, control through written laws and court actions, and the economic dependence of all government services.

Discursive limits

- As discussed in Volume 4, language is the primary means we now use to change people and our situations (done through people).
- Language does not have effects from the words themselves but from the social relationships and reciprocities between the speakers, this means that in bad situations in which either resources or social relationships are not opportunities, then language will be ineffective or silenced.
- We can do less with language now to change our bad situations, except through strangers and written laws. People will still try from their histories of shaping others through language, but these will result in exaggerations and novel attempts. This predicts a large number of speech and thought 'disorders' in modern life (see Chapter 4 for more) and also a larger number of emotional and other non-word attempts to change the social relationships and resources (through social relationships) in bad situations (V4.6).

Psychiatrists and clinical psychologists are not trained in using a 'sociological imagination' to see the societal effects acting on their individual clients and shaping their behaviours (Mills, 1959). All the above *societal sources of conflict and constraint*, which are much less obvious than the more local variety, are likely to lead more frequently to what are labelled as 'mental health' symptoms, because they are less likely to be observed and recognized.

For example, domestic violence is usually more observable and noticeable than 'institutional' violence, even when it is shaped by societal structures and barriers. So domestic violence perpetrators are less likely to be labelled with 'mental health' issues than those trying to do something to change their lives when it has been shaped by institutional violence (by lashing out at all of society)—because for the latter it will look like their responses are coming from 'within them and be attributed to internal issues'.

The societal bad situations arising from patriarchy, economics, etc. are also not tied to particular settings, people, or objects, which leads to a further problem. This means that the pressure or force from these bad situations is on the person *the whole time*, making the situation even worse, 24/7. The 'symptoms' (what has been shaped to try and change their bad situation) can then appear at any time or place and the actual setting is not important in understanding what is going on. People can cry, have panic attacks, or suddenly feel sad, and these might not be related to any of the immediate circumstances. You need to trace the bad situations they are in or have been in and how these are affecting all their other life contexts, and not to over-interpret the setting they happen to be in (Guerin, 2019).

But the basic point is that life has a lot of potential conflicts and stress, and when these occur people respond in whatever ways they have learned or with whatever is possible. If nothing is possible or no behaviours have been learned, then they will behave with almost random responses to these bad situations or else exaggerate any common behaviours that are available.

Bad situations and how they can affect language use: breaking down beliefs, reality, and identity

Being in bad situations does not only shape specific behaviours. If the bad situations mess up our social relationships, then this will mess up all our talking and thinking (V4.3, V4.4). This is not just about how we talk and tell stories to the people we know, but also messes up the way a lot of our lives are structured through our discourses to influence people (V5.6). The whole structuring, planning, and different versions of self-identity used to foster social relationships to gain resources, are also messed up. Our stories are broken and changed (V4.4, V4.7, V5.6) and this changes our resources. Even grammar can be affected (V5.2).

Here are some consequences to consider, again as a fairly abstract guide to sensitize readers, not to give an exhaustive list of how these bad situations alter the effects we can get from our language and our thinking:

- Our painful behaviours are *shaped by our contexts*, in which conflicts and problems occur, like any other behaviours, but the contexts in which we live have been changing over the last few centuries and especially over the last century, and achieving both resources and social relationships (mainly with strangers) in our lives now is more abstract, language-based, and difficult.

- We must remember that *the talk and discourses we construct around why we do all our behaviours does not cause or control those behaviours* (V4.4, V5.6). The talk and discourses are part of our social life, so a person with major life difficulties *should not be expected* to have discourses about what has happened to them. In this sense, *everyone's* talk, conversation, and discourse about why they do what they do is gratuitous and is only there to negotiate social relationships (although this is extremely important), not to 'cause' their behaviours; that is, these discourses do not control our behaviours.

- This means that if social relationships have been damaged from bad situations, and this is a collateral or direct effect of *most* bad situations, then the 'normal' (i.e. social) connections to reality (talk) will be loosened as well. The direct sense of 'reality' (V4.6) will not be affected (cf. Bleuler, 1911), meaning that walking around and seeing, and lifting chairs, etc. will usually still be fine. But so much of how we 'put' together reality and have *to talk about it as reality* is based on having social relationships to learn all this and then to talk about it. Despite being able to lift chairs, doing this action will usually occur under social relationship control and be subject to punishment, evaluation, needing explanations, etc. In terms of the Gestalt triangle (V4.1), we can still draw the accurate figure but our talk about a triangle or a mess of lines will be different.

- So, having a *disturbed sense of reality* can mean two very different things. Almost all of Bleuler's descriptions of 'schizophrenia', for example, are about talking and discourses and the person having only weak control over these. All the 'associations' and 'affectivity' are 'not connected to reality' but this refers to not being connected to the social/ discursive ways our realities are 'packaged' in terms of consistency, plans, goals, stories, justifications, coherence, grammar, etc., and not to walking around and not treading on the cat.

- Basically, *if bad situations lead to a major loss of social relationships then our social/discursive reality will suffer*, not just relationship activities. Various symptoms relate to this occurrence (hearing voices, dissociation, etc.), but they are held together by weak social relationships, not by a brain disease. This will majorly affect how beliefs are presented, self-identity talk, and social relationships when language does not function.

- What is really needed here is for the reader to get a strong sense of how their own 'normal' reality as experienced is held together by *social/ discursive relationships through social and societal control* and especially including language patterns and stories (V5.6). This is through the patterns of language use; the flow of language itself and how it appears to others; the (discursive) consistencies expected between all you do (actions, talking, and thinking); giving appearances of coherence; the 'me' thoughts'; giving the impression of everything being under your own control; being able to explain what you are doing to others; what you attend to and look at; how your gaze moves and focuses; being able to justify and explain whatever actions you do; responding appropriately (Bleuler's 'associations'); and making every associative or emotional response relate to the ongoing flow of activities and interactions.

- For those painful behaviours that have an obvious contextual origin (financial problems, grief from a loss, violence from someone known), there are professionals who can help with the pain and suffering and work to change the contexts (and sometimes, even in modernity, your family and community can still help with these) and *the discourses and stories will be patched up concurrently* (V5.6). Part of what therapy does is to create or rehearse your discourses to explain things to others.

- For painful behaviours that seem to have *no* obvious contextual origin, some are problems with relationships and resources that have occurred over a long time, and that *have accrued a lot of new discourses around them*, but the problems can be identified and solved with the parties involved and stories provided to suit.

- For other painful behaviours, when there seems to be *no* obvious contextual origin, the person has no idea what is shaping their behaviours, *has no talk initially around the behaviours*, is not fitting in with life and the behaviours just appear, or if the behaviour becomes locked into the context and becomes chronic, *then stories will start to be built around what seems to be going on but these might not relate to the actual source of the bad situation*. Wild stories can be produced.

- Some of these painful behaviours that seem to have no obvious contextual origin will be due to the person having their life *shaped by events outside of their control,* but that cannot be seen (e.g. lack of opportunities, gender, poverty, societal oppression) so the problem is not obvious and *no discourses are possible other than fictional or pretending that everything is all right.*

- With a contextual approach to emotional behaviours (V4.6), all these inexplicable sufferings that seem to come from nowhere will generate a number of *potentially random behaviours* if a response is required in the social context in which the person lives.

- To change the painful behaviour, *we need to help change the person's contexts* as far as this is possible. If they are stuck with poor opportunities or constraints that are backed by the whole of society, such as patriarchal or colonization constraints on behaviour, this will be difficult and other solutions might be needed to avert these societal contexts rather than remove them completely.

- Finally, in Chapters 1 and 2 (and V5.6) I argued that in life we mostly assume (wrongly) that 'we' *are* our main talk and thinking, and that this talk and thinking controls what we do. Earlier, I gave reasons why this seems to be perfectly true for everyday life, even though our talk and thinking are really there to negotiate social relationships afterwards and not control what we do. Armed with all this, you need to remember that for someone who has painful behaviours that seem to have no obvious contextual origin, *on top of everything else* they will also be very scared, since their normal 'we' or 'me' discourses have disappeared and they seem no longer in control, or are at least *dissociated* from everything around them. This can lead to new 'symptoms' but means that in general they will be uncertain and worried about what is happening to them. For example, those who have learned discourses about always trying to be in control might have overly aggressive beliefs that they tell you without wanting them challenged.

The Power Threat Meaning Framework approach

To finish, I would like to give a brief outline and endorsement of a very similar approach, the Power Threat Meaning Framework (PTMF; Johnstone et al., 2018). The main differences to the present approach are really in emphasis and current focus rather than anything of substance. Both agree that 'mental health' symptoms do not arise from any sort of disease but are responses to bad external situations (I have been calling these 'bad situations' whereas they use the term 'threats'). They also agree on the futility of the DSM approach to diagnosis, and on the need to focus our understanding of a person on their *situation,* as partly done in 'psychological formulations' (Johnstone, 2018; Johnstone et al., 2018).

In terms of the bad situations leading to the dysfunctional responses to threats, the PTMF starts with fundamental inequalities in society (my 'opportunities') and the ideological meanings (my 'discourses') that support those. These lead to increases (through no fault of the person) in levels of *insecurity*, lack of *social cohesion, mistrust,* violence and conflict, *prejudice, discrimination,* and social relationship issues across societies (all consequences of stranger relationships). These are said to lead to disruptions in early *childhood attachments* (weakening of familial relationships by stranger relationships), which increases the risk of adverse ('bad') situations.

Without denying the substance of what the PTMF is trying to say, these discourses are very much internal explanations that border on causation (Pathway 1, response 3), and the present book's approach merely wishes to analyse these *further* into the material bases of life that are no longer being achieved in such bad situations (Pathway 2). This is a change in wording and contextualization, not of substance.

As an example of *childhood attachment,* the present approach would do more analysis of the modern societal replacement of familial relations with stranger relationships even while being raised in a family (babysitters, schools, kindergarten), and how this can lead to poor relations within families and increased risk of abuse. These problems also get exacerbated because they change other contexts that might have been unrelated otherwise (as Figure 3.1 tries to illustrate). We need to apply a sociological imagination to childhood attachment, not treat it as an internal thing.

So, some of the PTMF discourses are still essentially 'internal' and use everyday language, that people 'naturally' are seeking 'meaning' in life, whereas the present approach covers the same ground but with the material world of people getting resources through social relationships—resource–social relationship pathways. This was the third of the Pathway 1 responses to the Gestalt problem (V4.1), and the PTMF also does a bit of the first response—using brain explanations.

The PTMF's current work also focuses more than the present approach on how early childhood threats lead to later 'mental health' effects, but without enough emphasis (from this book's perspective) on how those awful childhood experiences actually change and limit the child's many other contexts *at the time,* and how these contextual changes (more than just the original bad events) lead forward to the later 'symptoms'. The PTMF also currently focuses less on the *hidden* nature of contexts from which 'mental health' symptoms arise, and therefore with less detailed analysis of the *societal* constraints of economics, patriarchy, etc., which produce bad situations that cannot be easily seen.

But these are all minor changes in focus and future directions rather than anything substantial, and there no doubt will be convergence as both these frameworks are developed more and applied in real cases.

Another difference is that of the PTMF use of 'threat' and the related common term in social work and elsewhere of 'trauma-based' situations. I agree with them that threat and trauma situations are what I call 'bad situations', but my only difference is to give equal time to the other bad situations that can lead to problems in behaviour but that do not resemble 'threats' or 'trauma' in the usual meanings of these words (Sweeney & Taggart, 2018). I also emphasize that many behaviours are produced from threats or trauma, including crime and bullying, and that 'mental health' behaviours are on a continuum with these and not a distinct category.

Poverty and most of the societal bad situations do not appear in life as would be described by the words 'threat' or 'trauma', mainly because their effects are hidden and disguised, and sometimes even *made* to appear 'normal' and non-threatening (and people frequently get blamed for being poor!). Patriarchy could certainly be considered in the long run as a threat to women and could be perceived by many as being traumatic, since so many behaviours are often restricted and controlled out of women's reach, therefore restricting many solutions to their problems. But these bad effects of patriarchy happen over time and there is no single threat or traumatic *event* as such. Also, the male–female differences have developed community discourses that they are 'natural' or normal', making them look less like 'traumatic' events, even though the actual cumulative effects can be just as devastating.

So, I merely want to add *more* bad situations rather than take away the ones covered by these groups, which are important and sadly pervasive, and I wish to link them with other behaviours arising from these bad situations that are not even called 'mental health' behaviours. If people trying to help end up only focusing on or looking for those situations that might be described as a threat or a trauma with a 'psychological' outcome, then much will be missed. Early childhood abuse does lead to later 'mental health' issues (Johnstone et al., 2018), but it can also lead to a life of violence and crime or social withdrawal, which are bad but not often treated because they are not classified as 'mental health' problems. I want to be more inclusive of *all* the bad life effects of such events.

The key to the PTMF, then, is that responding to these threats is difficult, and therefore results in 'mental health' symptoms that are difficult to fathom and get medically pathologized. This happens because the threats compound, are hidden in societal practices and ideologies (discourses), and Western professionals are trained to see 'individual' problems. All this fits well with the present analysis.

The PTMF also nicely spells out in better detail than I have done here several specific groups and their common cluster of threats and threat responses (bad situations, like Table 3.2): children and young people, people with intellectual disabilities, older adults with cognitive impairments, and people with neurological impairments. They also detail common patterns for specific threats: threats to identities; surviving rejection, entrapment, and invalidation; surviving disrupted attachments and adversities as a child/ young person; surviving separation and identity confusion; surviving defeat, entrapment, disconnection, and loss; surviving social exclusion, shame, and coercive power; and surviving single threats. The present approach would emphasize more that problems with 'identities' are really problems with the full resource–social relationship pathways and how we present ourselves in our discourses, not something 'internal' (V5.5). (The next chapter will also briefly present the responses to threats that are suggested, as done here, to be the source of the 'mental health' symptoms.)

Conclusion: social actions for change

As mentioned earlier in this chapter, we should not be studying, analysing, or working with 'mental health' behaviours as if they were categorially separate from other human responses to bad situations. We should be working with *all behaviours shaped by bad situations in life* and not just the one set of these that occur when the bad situations cannot be observed easily. This changes our notions of intervention: any intervention should now focus on *changing a person's bad worlds, environments, or contexts* as paramount, although changing the societally produced bad situations is difficult (see Chapters 7 and 8). It shows why we need to shift and include *social and community action and activism* as part of the therapy or 'treatment' for 'mental health' (Guerin & Guerin, 2012), since it can help fix the bad situations.

We need to bring together all the experts who can help people solve any bad situations of life, regardless of the painful behaviours that emerge from this—whether crime, drugs, or the behaviours labelled as schizophrenia 'symptoms', etc. And by experts I do not mean just professionals—we need to learn from those with lived experience as well.

For example, if we seriously want to reduce generalized anxiety and depression in young people, we need to change how our societies are run and consider the effects of capitalism, patriarchy, bureaucracy, state power, etc. They are the abstract societal shapers of such 'generalized' effects (see Chapters 4 and 7). There are two problems, however, with trying to change the wider community and society as 'mental health' interventions:

1. *Currently most legal systems in any part of the world hold 'individuals' responsible for what they do, say, and think, with only a few exceptions.* Your history and environment are played down, as are the circumstances of your birth in legal cases. So, while we might observe and discover the contextual basis for the behaviours arising, this currently cannot be used in most societal systems as absolving the persons of legal responsibility.

2. *Many times the bad situations are, in fact, created by the society itself, and its rules, laws, way of enforcing rules and laws, and economic system.* Many people in Western capitalist societies do not want the sort of life you are forced to live in such a system. They feel like they have 'never fitted in with things' and did not choose to be born into such systems but have almost no alternatives except to try and live what are often called 'alternative lifestyles', and put up with it. As shown elsewhere (V5.3, V3), it is thought that a lot of the currently rising problems labelled 'generalized anxiety' and 'generalized depression' are responses to the strictures and restrictions of late capitalism. Avoidance by entertainment and excesses are increasingly prevalent and shaped by these bad situations.

References

Bleuler, E. (1911). *Dementia praecox or the group of schizophrenias.* New York, NY: International Universities Press.

Bovin, M. J., & Marx, B. P. (2011). The importance of the peritraumatic experience in defining traumatic stress. *Psychological Bulletin, 137,* 47–67.

Cohen, S. (Ed.) (1971). *Images of deviance.* London: Penguin.

Cohen, S., & Taylor, L. (1976). *Escape attempts: The theory and practice of resistance to everyday life.* London: Allen Lane.

Decker, S. H., & van Winkle, B. (1996). *Life in the gang: Family, friends, and violence.* New York, NY: Cambridge University Press.

Dembo, T., & Hanfmann, E. (1935). The patient's psychological situation upon admission to a mental hospital. *American Journal of Psychology, 47,* 381–408.

Eckert, P. (1989). *Jocks and burnouts: Social categories and identity in the high school.* New York, NY: Teachers College Press.

Glasper, I. (2006). *The day the country died: A history of anarcho punk 1980 to 1984.* London: Cherry Red Books.

Guerin, B. (2004). *Handbook for analyzing the social strategies of everyday life.* Reno, NV: Context Press.

Guerin, B. (2016). *How to rethink human behavior: A practical guide to social contextual analysis.* London: Routledge.

Guerin, B. (2017). *How to rethink mental illness: The human contexts behind the labels.* London: Routledge.

Guerin, B. (2019). What do therapists and clients talk about when they cannot explain behaviours? How Carl Jung avoided analysing a client's environments by inventing theories. *Revista Perspectivas em Análise Comportamento, 10,* 76–97.

Guerin, B., & Guerin, P. (2012). Re-thinking mental health for Indigenous Australian communities: Communities as context for mental health. *Community Development Journal, 47*(4), 555–570.

Haley, J. (1973). *Uncommon therapy: The psychiatric techniques of Milton H. Erickson, M.D.* London: Norton.

Hartman, S. (2017). *Wayward lives, beautiful experiments: Intimate histories of riotous black girls, troublesome women, and queer radicals.* New York, NY: W. W. Norton.

Johnstone, L. (2018). Psychological formulation as an alternative to psychiatric diagnosis. *Journal of Humanistic Psychology, 58*, 30–46.

Johnstone, L., Boyle, M., Cromby, J., Dillon, J., Harper, D., Kinderman, P., ... Read, J. (2018). *The Power Threat Meaning Framework: Towards the identification of patterns in emotional distress, unusual experiences and troubled or troubling behaviour, as an alternative to functional psychiatric diagnosis.* Leicester, UK: British Psychological Society.

Maté, G. (2009). *In the realm of hungry ghosts: Close encounters with addiction.* London: Vintage.

Mills, C. W. (1959). *The sociological imagination.* Oxford: Oxford University Press.

Nordhoff, C. (1875/1966). *The communistic societies of the United States: From personal visit and observation.* New York, NY: Dover.

Orwell, G. (1933). *Down and out in Paris and London.* London: Victor Gollancz.

Qi, R., Palmier-Claus, J., Simpson, J., Varese, F., & Bentall, R. (2019). Sexual minority status and symptoms of psychosis: The role of bullying, discrimination, social support, and drug use: Findings from the Adult Psychiatric Morbidity Survey 2007. *Psychology and Psychotherapy: Theory, Research and Practice, 93*, 1–17.

Riggs, D. W., & Treharne, G. J. (2017) Decompensation: A novel approach to accounting for stress arising from the effects of ideology and social norms. *Journal of Homosexuality, 64*, 592–605.

Rowe, P. (2018). *Heavy metal youth identities: Researching the musical empowerment of youth transitions and psychosocial wellbeing.* London: Emerald Publishing.

Sartwell, C. (2014). *How to escape: Magic, madness, beauty, and cynicism.* New York, NY: Excelsior Editions.

Sweeney, A., & Taggart, D. (2018). (Mis)understanding trauma-informed approaches in mental health. *Journal of Mental Health, 27*, 383–387.

Truong, F. (2018). *Radicalized loyalties: Becoming Muslim in the West.* London: Polity.

Wyatt-Brown, B. (1988). The mask of obedience: Male slave psychology in the old South. *American Historical Review, 93*, 1228–1252.

Yablonsky, L. (1962). *The violent gang.* London: Penguin.

4 Contextualizing 'mental health' symptoms without diagnoses

Initial explorations

From the first chapters we have got to a point that clearly puts the focus on solving the bad situations in people's lives, how to contextually ana-lyse these situations (Guerin, 2016), and how to change them, regardless of whether these bad situations have shaped the DSM-listed behaviours or others, such as violence, bullying, lying and exploitation, domestic vio-lence, excessive or dependent drug taking, exiting, self-harm, 'criminal' behaviours, etc. This also means that all the people currently working sep-arately on these 'problem' behaviours arising from similar bad situations can now work together better, regardless of their historically labelled 'dis-ciplines' (e.g. social workers, psychologists, police, etc.). We should now be looking for 'experts' in analysing and changing specific types of bad situations, instead of experts in specific 'problem' behaviours. And experts include people with first-hand experience of living in such bad situations, not just professionals.

Some bad situations, however, are difficult to observe and to change, and many of these are shaped by societal structures that will need changing in order to help the individual, even if this is difficult to accomplish. So, getting to the full contexts for 'mental health' and other behaviours will need new types of observation (V2.1), analysis (V2), and intervention (Guerin, 2005), and a strong 'sociological imagination' (Mills, 1959). But the focus should now be on *finding ways to analyse and change bad situations as they arise in people's lives, regardless of the specific 'problem' behaviours that might have been shaped over time* (Fromene & Guerin, 2014; Fromene, Guerin, & Krieg, 2014; Guerin, 2019; Guerin & Guerin, 2012; Ryan, Guerin, Elmi, & Guerin, 2019).

The purpose of this chapter is to look more closely at just those behaviours listed in the DSM and make suggestions for how bad life situations might have shifted them from being ordinary behaviours to become exaggerated, the only behaviours available, and getting locked into life so as to become chronic. This again is intended as a way of shaping the reader to become sensitized and begin to observe such transformations occurring. This is not meant as any sort of exhaustive or definitive list of how this happens. And it is not a new DSM! Its only purpose is to sensitize readers so they begin focusing their attention on to the *bad situations shaping the DSM behaviours into their worst forms*. Stop looking inside the person for the answers and look instead more thoroughly into their messed-up life situations.

To do this I will work through nine groups of 'mental health' behaviours/ symptoms taken directly from the DSM, and for each of the behaviours I will suggest *possibilities* (V2) for how these might *function* as ordinary behaviours but then get reshaped by the bad situations of life given in the previous chapter, and how the exaggerated versions might be shaped and locked in. I will not look here at other behaviours shaped by bad situations such as violence and excessive or dependent drug use. That remains to be done.

In the previous two chapters (and V3), I have looked at the subtle and hidden lifeworlds, environments, or contexts for 'mental health' behaviours, and at the actual behaviours, talking, and thinking found in the DSM 'mental health' behaviours (V3). My task now is to show *possibilities* (V2) for how these might be functionally connected—how the DSM-listed behaviours might be shaped by bad environments and not by brain diseases or chemical imbalances. The shaping of behaviours from living in bad situations is certainly complex and differs according to even small changes in contexts (e.g. Wyatt-Brown, 1988), and we are now catching up on 60 years of missed opportunities (V4.1). So what is written here *are only possiblities to consider*, and analyses should carefully follow observations of personal contexts of real cases, rather than what is set out here. Every case and every life will differ.

From this, the goal is to explore how we might begin observing these 'hidden' functional connections between bad situations and the behaviours, but done *without the DSM groupings*, and then how we might *change the bad environments* to improve people's lives (see Chapters 5–8). They are meant to sensitize readers and practitioners to the *possible* ways our societal and subtle *external* contexts of life shape the behaviours that are currently labelled 'mental health' issues, remembering from the last chapter that many *other* behaviours are shaped by bad situations, but that arbitrarily do not get help from the same professionals. The proof will be in whatever use *you*, as the reader, make of these suggestions to see the way your clients, friends, or yourself, are being shaped. This will probably not be in ways exactly mentioned in this book, but I hope the sensitization process will assist you to observe them in new ways.

With social contextual analysis (Guerin, 2016; Mills, 1959) you should be able to see an individual in distress and go into their world, participate if you can, and see the observable conflicts and problems *in their worlds*

(Pathway 2). Simultaneously, you should be able to 'see' the *societal and discursive contexts* that are structuring their bad situation (as sociologists, sociolinguists, and social anthropologists have learned to do), even though these are hidden to most people. Psychiatrists and psychologists in particular need to learn to 'see' through these societal lenses. They have not been trained to do this and miss most of what is going on, and cover this up by explaining it as something originating 'inside' the person (Pathway 1).

What are the 'mental health' behaviours?

The question we get to next is, which 'mental health' behaviours are shaped, when, and from what bad situations or contexts? Are they arbitrary or tightly controlled by specific circumstances? Are there patterns? Are there groupings from having similar environments?

In general, it seems that the 'mental health' behaviours that emerge from bad situations depend a lot on *what behaviours are available* in any of the bad situations, but perhaps within the availability they are arbitrary and also changing more than currently theorized. People are trying to deal with, survive, or escape from bad situations they probably do not understand, and there is no assumption in this that they are shaped into only one single behaviour.

From the DSM and psychiatric perspective, the brain diseases of 'mental illness' lead to specific and unique behaviours that should not change over time except to get more extreme (from brain degeneration). But from a contextual approach, people might be shaped to do many different responses over time and change. In reality, this change, flexibility, and variability for individuals over time, is currently *hidden* within the DSM by the following:

• The large range of comorbidities, which cannot be ignored under the pretence that they are independent diagnoses just because the DSM says so.
• The huge overlap in actual symptoms between 'independent' disorders that are diagnoses (now revealingly called 'transdiagnostic' symptoms), which is 'corrected' by a large listing of 'differential diagnoses'.
• The fact that those diagnosing with the DSM often change diagnoses or dispute diagnoses, whereas this can occur *both* because the client's actual behaviours *have* changed over time and because the diagnoses are not a good category system.
• The apathy of institutions and individuals to actually look closely into the client's worlds.

I just don't think that psychiatric diagnoses are the same as diagnoses like 'broken pelvis' and 'arthritis'. I've been given different diagnoses at different times in my life, simply because I was dealing with different issues and was distressed in different ways ... just like anyone else would be.

(Broug, 2008, p. 39)

What this chapter will try and do is to present some ways that the 'psychiatric symptoms' might be shaped more specifically by bad situations. I believe that *the rigidity of the DSM approach has covered up a lot more flexibility than is realized* for people in bad situations trying to find new ways to behave so as to change or escape that situation, especially if we include those other outcomes of bad situations not defined as 'mental health' issues, such as bullying, exploitation, and 'criminal' activities.

When we break finally from the DSM, we will find that people are not stagnant in their 'mental disorders' but are much more flexible to change and adapt as opportunities and their situations vary. The distinction made between 'mental health' and *other* behaviours arising from bad situations will also disappear and we can focus on changing the bad situations regardless of what they have produced. Drug treatments are likely to 'stabilize symptoms' because they limit the changes in the person's world by making them not want to attempt anything new.

Like most of the books in this series, others have suggested similar ideas from which I have learned. Meyer, for example, wrote about 'substitute reactions': "Such a reaction is *a faulty response or substitution of an insufficient or protective or evasive or mutilated attempt at adjustment*" (Meyer, 1948, p. 199, italics in original). The basic idea is similar, that there are bad situations and the person is trying to deal with them, but most alternative or 'normal' ways are blocked so something else is shaped. But I see the new behaviours not just as *substitutes* for the 'proper' behaviour, and certainly not as 'faulty' given the bad circumstances, but as being (1) shaped or sampled from what is possible within the person's bad life circumstances, (2) not substituted from elsewhere, (3) not necessarily functional to 'solve' the whole bad situation but perhaps parts of it, and (4) probably with multiple *different* attempts being made, especially over time when one attempt is not working. Another related group of literature focuses on bad situations that were defined as 'frustrating' situations, which not only produced aggression but a range of other responses (see Barker, Dembo, & Lewin, 1941/1976; de Rivera, 1976; Sears, 1941).

For example, in the worst-case scenarios in which *all* social relationships are blocked and alternatives are not possible, what can a person even do (cf. Wyatt-Brown, 1988)? One could use *breathing* and *moving* to try and alter the events going on around you, or at least as distraction or avoidance, and self-harm is almost always a possible behaviour in even very bad situations to try and change the social relationship contexts in some way. (Children sometimes try holding their breath to change their bad situation, but this does not work for long.)

Unfortunately, forms of violence and bullying are always available, physical or verbal, but not always successful. Social anthropologists have found that food and eating are often more about social relationships than nutrition (Guerin, 1992), and changing something about their *eating* and *food patterns* is often a tactic people use in a bad situation in an attempt to change it, if there are no other options available. You can also still *speak* and *make other sounds*, and even though in the bad situation they will not change things in the normal way that language use does, they can be used for attempts at changing the bad situation. You can also then *exaggerate* all the possibilities above, which might change your situation somewhat, but although this might work initially (people take notice or avoid you) it runs the risk of causing further problems. And you can always withdraw, both physical withdrawal (many variations including depressive symptoms) and verbal withdrawal (including dissociation), albeit with consequences.

What you then notice is that forms of these 'always available behaviours' appear throughout the DSM, especially in bad situations in which the person is locked into it, alternative behaviours have no effect on changing the person's bad situation, and our normal language methods of persuasion are not working. And they also form common behaviours *in other bad situations* (Wyatt-Brown, 1988). It is not that they are 'transdiagnostic'; it is that the diagnosis itself is faulty.

Contextualizing the DSM behaviours

Elsewhere (Guerin, 2017, chap. 4) I have approached this question by going to the latest edition of the DSM and cutting and pasting all the behaviours listed under the main diagnostic criteria for all the major 'disorders'. While these all have provisos attached to them to be diagnosed as 'mental health' issues rather than normal forms of some behaviour, such as being intense, leading to non-functional outcomes, and being chronic over certain periods of time (all of which are fairly arbitrary), that is irrelevant to what I am doing here. I want to examine all the behaviours themselves that are used for diagnosis and to look for the circumstances that shape them normally and then make suggestions as to how they might be shaped in exceptionally bad situations to try and change or escape the bad conditions.

This first involved reading a lot of books written about 'mental health' *before* the DSM era. One side effect of diagnosis has been that most mental health research and writing no longer focuses on describing individual behaviours/symptoms and their contexts but focuses strongly instead only on the diagnostic clusters. This means that we now get very few research descriptions of what a person actually does and thinks, and the contexts for these, and much more theories about whether what they are doing fits into a named diagnostic cluster (Pathway 1). The DSM has produced a narrowed vision in 'mental health' thinking and research. Despite their problems, the older books (pre-DSM) frequently gave lots of examples and case studies with as much context as they could of the person's life situation, and they thought beyond just squeezing what was seen into a DSM category. In the words of C. M. Campbell (1925, p. 11): "I ask you, therefore, to consider our topic to be not 'mental disorders', but men, women, and children in difficulty, suffering, hoping, thwarted, groping."

Luckily, there is also a growing and useful literature of the experiences coming from people with first-hand experience and from their carers. These were all used to suggest possibilities of contexts for the raw DSM-listed behaviours. Some useful volumes were: Bleuler, 1911/1950, 1912; Broug, 2008; Cameron & Magaret, 1951; Cleckley, 1964; Costello, 1970; Dorman, 2006; #Emerging Proud, 2019; Factora-Borchers, 2014; Janet, 1902, 1907; Johnstone et al., 2018; Jung, 1960; Longden, Corstens, Escher, & Romme, 2012; Meyer, 1948; Rogers & Leydesdorff, 2004; Romme, Escher, Dillon, Corstens, & Morris, 2009; Schilder, 1950, 1976; Schneider, 2010; Sullivan, 1973, 1974; Watson, 2019; Xinran, 2002.

So, this is the material I will work with here (cf. Guerin, 2017, chap. 4). After pulling out all the behaviours (actions, talking, and thinking) from the main DSM categories, I found, like others have, that there were a lot of repetitions and 'transdiagnostic' behaviours. This appears in the descriptions themselves, without even taking into account the very long outlines of (1) how to avoid confusing similar-looking behaviours ('differential diagnoses'), or (2) the comorbidity patterns that are also extensive (these two raise questions as to whether the DSM diagnoses are at all 'scientific'; no other taxonomic classification system would survive such vagaries).

I ignored the differential diagnoses and vague separations into comorbidity patterns because we are now looking at the original shaping of concrete actions, ways of talking, and ways of thinking, and those extra conditions (differential diagnoses and comorbidities) are only there to support the biologically baseless *groupings* of the symptoms into 'disorders', and do not add anything to our understanding of the behaviours themselves (in fact, they detract from our trying to understand the occurrences of these behaviours by focusing people on the labelling). This becomes clear if you look at the alphabetical list of DSM symptoms, stripped from their fictional 'disorder' groupings (Guerin, 2017, table 4.4). They are just a bunch of normal behaviours that can go wrong when shaped and exaggerated in bad situations.

From all these DSM behaviours, I (re)grouped the symptoms into the following nine new groups based upon their *functional relations with bad environments* (Guerin, 2017). (All the actual behaviours from the DSM will be listed later in this chapter so no information has been lost with my groupings, and another grouping could be created if the reader wishes to try that.)

1. Very general behaviours.
2. General changes to mood presentation.
3. Actions unusual.
4. Social relationships problematic.
5. Thinking and talking problematic: general.
6. Thinking and talking problematic: specific.
7. Thinking and talking problematic: identity talk.
8. Thinking and talking problematic: talking about social relationships.
9. Thinking and talking problematic: anxiety and fear.

In presenting them here, as will become clear I hope, it made more sense to put these nine into *three groupings that share a lot of real-life functional or shaping properties* (notice that I have kept the original numbering in this new ordering here and in what follows):

Group 1: general behaviours

1. Very general behaviours.
2. General changes to mood presentation.
3. Actions unusual.
5. Thinking and talking problematic: general.

Group 2: social behaviours

4. Social relationships problematic.
8. Thinking and talking problematic: talking about social relationships.

Group 3: language and discourse issues

6. Thinking and talking problematic: specific.
7. Thinking and talking problematic: identity talk.
9. Thinking and talking problematic: anxiety and fear.

There are similar functional possibilities within each group (that was how they were chosen) so some initial summaries will also occur for each of the three big groups looked at over all the individual 'symptoms' within that group.

In reading through the following, I would like readers to again be clear that this is not about a 'scientific' discourse of putting the one truth about the symptoms into new boxes. My aim is a practical one of breaking down the rigidity with which we currently 'observe' these behaviours and now learn to 'see' the possible contexts at the same time we 'see' the behaviours. Most professionals at the moment only 'observe' actual behaviours to try and 'see' DSM diagnoses, and they usually only observe verbal reports of behaviours. They need to directly 'see' all the possible contexts for the behaviours that have been shaped.

I am deliberately trying to reshape the reader into seeing these 'mental health' behaviours in new ways that follow Pathway 2 (V4.1). My aim is not for you to believe all the following but for professionals and others to observe clients in new ways, to 'see' their behaviours *and their contexts* with your new 'sociological imagination'. The details are meant to give possibilities to break up the current rigid forms of observation and analysis that focus solely on establishing diagnoses as if that was the end point of all this.

Group 1: general behaviours

In this section I discuss possibilities for the specific DSM symptoms (actions, talking, and thinking) that were grouped under my four subheadings of *general behaviours*. They are meant to break the behaviours into functional groups, that is, behaviours that might function in similar ways in many (bad) contexts and might even be substitutable (which potentially could be useful for building new interventions). These are my constructions, however, so they can be ignored for the finer behaviours that are taken from the DSM, or you might construct your own, new categories. In the long run, any broader categories should be described from good functional participatory research with real people coping with bad situations, rather than my 'possibility' approach here (Guerin, 2016, 2018; Guerin, Leugi, & Thain, 2018).

Preamble: what does being 'general' tell us?

Before looking at the details, it is worth saying something about the whole 'general' category I have imposed. In calling them 'general', all of these involve *behaviours that are not tied closely to specific situations*. Just this alone can indicate the following:

- The bad situation(s) are likely to have been shaped through the *broad, societal contexts* that can affect a person's whole life but which cannot easily be controlled: patriarchy, poverty, capitalism and neoliberalism, race or oppression. These behaviours are not maintained in just one or another specific situations of life, and so these 'general' behaviours can appear 'unexpectedly' in situations where they might seem inappropriate. While a traumatic event such as being in a car crash might in the short term only show symptoms in or near cars, the behaviours in this group are effects that can occur more generally. Even in 'inappropriate' or 'irrelevant' contexts, the painful general contexts are still present in the person's life. They have also not gone away even if the person gets distracted for short periods.

- If related to *social relationships*, the problem is likely to have arisen from important or frequent social relationships not going well, especially where there are many resource interdependencies within those relationships. In such situations, all pathways become inaccessible if resources are tied to strongly dependent social relationships. That is, some will apply to mainly family relationships where a lot is at stake, especially if young or not independent.

- For *talking and thinking*, the behaviours in this 'general' grouping indicate contextually that the audiences shaping and maintaining such patterns are broad, not about single people, and are probably abstract audiences such as 'social norms', verbal groups such as 'men', or any forms of public media. These are not bad situations tied to a single specific audience.

- While there might be a limited situation as an *originating event*, frequently such events affect a person's life context very broadly afterwards, so there still is a general effect. For example, while abuse from one person is very specific, the effects from this in some (most?) cases is general as well ("What if *someone* found out this happened? What would *they* think of me?").

- General behaviours can also be *'emotional' responses* to situations in which the person does not know *how* to respond (especially when it is not shaped by a single specific situation) and yet a response is demanded (V4.6). If specific people were shaping the bad situations there would be specific behaviours required and non-language emotional responses would usually occur only within those specific situations, not in general. In these cases, general behaviours can be shaped that might reappear in unexpected new 'emotional situations' (V4.6).

Someone might start crying or get angry in seemingly 'irrelevant' or 'inappropriate' situations.

- The person's behaviours might have been shaped in a very *restricted life-world* so that there have been few alternatives learned; their behaviours have been shaped to occur across *most* of their (albeit restricted) life domains so they have not learned more specific responding across more varied settings.

- One problem from this group is that because these general behaviours do not depend on a specific setting or 'stimulus' for their occurrence, this means *they are a constant pressure on a person* regardless of time of day or place, and the attempts at adaptive behaviours can occur in non-specific places and times.

- This therefore means that *when* and *where* these behaviours occur will not tell you anything useful about the behaviour and its functioning in that person's world, and so these factors should not be over-interpreted; this includes symptoms currently linked to the categories of depression, panic attacks, generalized anxiety, and crying.

If we look now at the four 'general' subgroups and the specific DSM behaviours within each grouping, the possibilities are also very broad. The functional or strategic uses of these behaviours are far more subtle and complex within real contexts. For example, they have sometimes been characterized as, "move against people, move towards people, and move away from people" (Horney), "voice, loyalty, and exit" (Hirschman), or the inevitable "fight and flight", but these words do not get us far. These sound like we know something, but without the contexts we know nothing, and when we know the specific contexts those slogans are no use anyway.

1. Very general behaviours

These are behaviours that will function in different ways across many different life contexts as ways of (originally, at least) attempting to cope with bad or threatening situations—they are not a response to a specific bad situation. It is important to note for these behaviours and the ones to follow in this grouping that the actual functioning cannot be gleaned by the form or topography of the behaviours, they always need contextualizing: we can cry from sadness or from happiness so crying by itself tells us little. The 'general behaviours' group is probably the most difficult for this since they can occur in many contexts, so neither the form or topography of the behaviour itself, nor when and where it occurs, tell us much, and interpreting these should be avoided. Only engaging with the person's worlds can tell us about the actual functioning (Guerin, 2018).

So, the main point, going back to the ideas of emotions (V4.6), is that the 'symptoms' seen are probably almost random responses to a very bad general life situation for which there were no clear or more obvious responses that would have changed this situation (how do you fight patriarchy on your own?), or to change a generally bad lifeworld in which nothing is working for any sort of resource–social relationship pathway—the person simply does not 'fit in' with life. In both cases *the 'symptom' should not be over-interpreted* since it could be almost random.

For example, we have seen above that in the absence of any other responses that might affect or change a person's bad lifeworld, eating, sleeping, body pains, breathing, negative symptoms, violence, catatonia, and abstract discourses unrelated to the real world are a few of the minimal responses left for people to vary and exaggerate, to try and make changes in their world. *These are all responses that can be done in the absence of any resources or supportive social relationships*, so the person will be shaped to change these from 'normal' versions (e.g., the strong social relationship effects of constantly changing eating patterns, or ignoring good eating habits) and exaggerate if the situation does not change (which then becomes the DSM 'dysfunctional' eating habits). We can always be violent to change things, we can always affect people with strong and 'bullying beliefs' about abstract conspiracies or events that cannot be checked (although most of these will not be classified as 'mental health' issues).

Note how the normal interpretations of 'trying to get attention' or 'attention-seeking' fit in here. If you solely focus on social relationships then these behaviours can *look like* the person is trying to get attention, but this interpretation is not very helpful. The functional question then merely becomes, "Why do they even want attention?" (often answered weakly by appealing to abstract theories once again—"It is a natural human urge to make attachments and bond with people", Pathway 1).

The view here is that people are trying to change their bad situation and getting attention is almost always a first step in any change, since we need good social contexts for almost everything we need in life (resources). If you focus instead on the resource–social relationship pathways, then the person is not trying to get social attention or social attachment per se but *social exchanges* or interrelationships to build a new resource world *through* some forms of social relationship, and that is what you should be contextualizing. They are in a bad situational world *in general* and nothing seems to be able to change in their current resource–social relationship pathways. So, they will be shaped to vary a 'generally available behaviour' and exaggerate to change the current bad exchanges or develop new exchanges through people. So just 'explaining' such behaviours as 'attention-seeking' does not answer anything nor help us develop alternative strategies with the persons involved. The better question is: what do they want from the attention to improve their world?

There are almost certainly exceptions but in general, time should not be spent on interpreting the 'meaning' or 'sign' of the particular behaviour in these groups, but focus more on the following:

- What the overwhelming, general, or bad situation is about and what other responses might help change their environment ("What has happened to you?").
- What resource–social relationship pathways are present and what the person's discourses say about these.
- The possible generalized audiences for these behaviours (generalized other, social norms, media, someone).
- Who requires that some sort of response be made at all? Where is that pressure coming from (it could be from therapists in fact)?

Given the nature of these painful behaviours that might seem to have no obvious contextual origin, it must also be remembered that at a certain point *all* talking responses might be ineffective and there are *no* 'appropriate' discursive responses to the painful life contexts for an individual that might help. Acknowledging this and finding other *non-talking* responses might be the best immediate action for the behaviours here (Guerin, 2019). Many people survive their bad situations by changing them (even slightly) through doing non-language behaviours (since language has not been any use to them in their bad situation)—emotional responses and emotional discourses, music, poetry, art, film, design, etc. Some find at least one resource–social relationship pathway through these non-language behaviours to 'fit in' with people in similar situations and thereby avoid the exaggerations (V5.6; Rowe, 2018; Rowe & Guerin, 2018) (see Box 4.1).

2. General changes to mood presentation

While moods are 'explained' in psychology as internal states that originate within us, for the approach here they have been shaped functionally *to do things to people* like most other behaviour. In particular, moods are social like language, in the sense that they only function to change the person's *social* environment. Moods do not function with objects nor with non-human animals except in a different way that is, in any case, unrelated to the 'mood' itself (we sometimes apply our moods to objects—yelling at your car when it does not work—but this does not change anything and might only have been shaped to affect any people watching you).

Box 4.1 The DSM behaviours corresponding to my grouping

Very general behaviours

- *Crying spells*: crying can function both to gain attention (which still needs further functional analysis, remember) and also to keep people away and so avoid bad situations. It is common as a reaction when not having any other response available (even talking; V4.6) but still needing to respond, so there are real but nuanced questions of "Who is the crying for?", "What bad situation is this for?", or "If your crying could change something in your world, what would it be doing?" We also cry when overwhelmingly happy or perplexed (overwhelming also means generalized), so it is related to other behaviours in this list. In essence, crying tells us little that is specific unless we can find (1) what the overwhelming or bad situation is about, (2), what other responses might be more helpful and why are they currently blocked, (3) who are the audiences for crying (they might be generalized others or societal), and (4) who requires that some sort of response be made at all.

- *Desperation*: this DSM category does not clearly specify any concrete behaviours but the behaviours meant are probably related to the same scenarios as for crying above. There is an overwhelmingly bad situation, a response is required but the person has none, and so a flurry of other desperate things is done instead. The same four questions as above for 'crying spells' therefore apply.

- *Feeling overwhelmed*: as for the above two points, there is a bad situation and the person does not have responses to change things, but they are required to respond so a verbal response of 'being overwhelmed' is given. The same four questions as for 'crying spells' apply.

- *Unable to adjust to a particular stressor*: this DSM category restates as above that the person does not have any responses that can deal with the bad situation so is resorting to behaviours that they can vary and test out. Nothing is working to change anything.

- *Being awake throughout the night, decreased sleep, sleeping troubles*: this is a dubious DSM 'behaviour' since many sorts of problems can lead to sleeplessness, not just those labelled 'mental health'. Sleeplessness in everyday life can also result from being overwhelmed in *positive* ways, so the symptom probably tells us little. Sleep does have social properties in that it can be a way of avoiding bad situations or relationships and does not need money or other resources to do it.

- *Disturbance of eating or eating-related behaviour*: eating is an essential everyday activity, so as a response to a bad situation it certainly will affect and perhaps change the social behaviour of many others, whether this is to engage with them more or less. Social anthropologists have shown that eating and foods are usually more related to social relationship negotiations than to nutrition (Guerin, 1992). The attempt to change the bad situations outweighs the negative consequences here in the shaping process (not the person's 'faulty decision-making').

- *Somatic changes that affect the individual's capacity to function*: somatic changes to the body are common and have a discursive advantage that they cannot be monitored or checked. For those already in weak positions of power, this is an easily defensible way to respond in bad situations when other more direct responses are not changing the bad situation. If talking and other discourses as methods of changing people and situations have been silenced from a weak position of power, somatic changes can be one way of attempting to change things. It probably changes very little but if there are few other alternatives it might be observed.

- *Spending less time with friends and family*: this tells us little since functionally it could be (1) responding to specific bad situations involving the friends and family or (2) a general withdrawal because nothing else is working for the person in any part of life and is unrelated to anything specific about the immediate people.

- *Staying home from work or school*: as above.

- *Negative symptoms*: again, withdrawing from activities can always be done, even without resources of any sort and without fruitful social relationships, so the negative symptoms are almost always available as options shaped to change or escape bad situations. The specific negative symptoms might even be random.

- *Attention-seeking*: attention is a resource in a general way because any method of changing a bad situation through social relationship requires attention. In itself, however, it might be of little analytic use since we still need to find out the bad situation and what attempts are being made to escape or change once attention is gained. If uses of talking are being silenced it might be necessary for attention-seeking strategies first.

- *Increased sex drive*: as above but more specific.
- *Increased alcohol and drug use*: once again, attempts to respond to bad situations and pain but in a general avoidance or escape way. These behaviours will usually mean that the person's bad situations are widespread in their life and not momentary. You need to find where the bad situations in the person's whole life are coming from, and why not other behaviours as per the above.

For mood presentations, therefore, we need to look at these behaviours as strategies (the person might not know this or be able to talk about this = unconscious) that are trying to deal with or change in any way possible a bad *social* situation, but *usually when words are not functioning* and persuasion does not work in the social relationships (V4.3, V4.7). This could arise from: different audiences who are operating with different or contradictory outcomes; people who are blocking access to 'resources' and not listening; having an abundance of stranger social relationships that have no commitment or obligation, so there is less persuasion possible; the person being punished or silenced in talking and other discourse (especially women being silenced or interrupted by men); or people for whom some parts of the relationship are working but not others, thus giving contradictory outcomes (see Box 4.2).

3. Actions unusual

These are placed together from the DSM merely because they stand out from 'normal' behaviour in a way that can be called 'purposeful', but that really means that in the past the behaviours (or less exaggerated forms) have been shaped to be functional to bring about some change in bad contexts. Some appear ritualized (like being overly dramatic), meaning, almost paradoxically, that they stand out by being ordinary patterns of behaviour done in a non-ordinary way or in non-ordinary contexts. This might function to restrict possible outcomes from the social environment when contradictory outcomes are occurring, because other people would be expected to respond in the ordinary way. If the person acted in the way the environment is demanding, there would be contradictory outcomes (some bad), so one of the ordinary behaviours is exaggerated (made dramatic).

The possibility is often not considered that many of these unusual actions can also function to *avoid* social situations rather than being 'attention-seeking'. Acting in exaggerated and potentially violent ways can not only bully people into changing contexts in the way wanted (see 'social

Box 4.2 The DSM behaviours corresponding to my grouping

General changes to mood presentation

- *Affective instability*: indicates that different 'mood' or non-language responses are being tried to change the bad situation. The affect could be changing for different audiences or for trying out new approaches to changing the social relationships.
- *Emotion disrupted from normal*: trying exaggerations to change the current range of social relationships. This suggests that the 'normal' use of 'moods' is not working, and the person is not fitting in. It is related to the next category of 'actions unusual'.
- *Empty mood*: similar to 'negative symptoms'. This is a form of withdrawal as a strategy, or because they have been punished for responding 'in general'.
- *Excessive emotionality*: exaggerated forms of 'doing something' to change social relationships through emotional displays.
- *Hopelessness*: a loose term that covers a wide range of behaviours similar to all those here.
- *Moodiness that is out of character*: could be due to new audiences in life or similar to all the above; may be using moods shaped by one audience in another social relationship.
- *Lack of enjoyment, loss of interest in pleasurable activities*: trying to either change the resources in life, the social relationships, or the current resource–social relationship pathways.
- *Restricted range of emotional expression*: variation on all the above, showing that the normal emotions and moods can be changed by withdrawing or exaggerating to effect some sort of change in life's bad situations.
- *Sad mood, sadness*: exaggerating non-language responding probably when all resource–social relationship pathways changed, and when language is not working to make changes in your world.

relationships problematic', p. 97), but in other situations they can also function just to have other people *exit* from the context and leave the protagonist alone. If you rant, exaggerate your speech, or have exaggerated hand and body movements, people will leave you alone. Try it. This is why behaviours need to be contextualized and not taken at face value (Guerin, 2016).

In many ways these can be viewed as the *physical* versions of the previous category, 'general changes to mood presentation', because they have similar functionality. Being more physical, however, they are likely to have more negative consequences from others and escalate into exaggeration more quickly. They are also more likely to *distract* from the bad situations rather than succeed as (misguided) attempts to change things (see Box 4.3).

Box 4.3 The DSM behaviours corresponding to my grouping

Actions unusual

- *Appear dramatic, emotional, or erratic*: the usual ways of changing your world are not working, with language or without, and these get shaped to be exaggerated or constantly varying, distractions, or to avoid future social interactions.

- *Appear odd or eccentric, eccentricities of behaviour*: as above, but not to get attention per se but to gain pathways for resources and social relationships, to provide a distraction, or to avoid future social interactions.

- *Disorganized or abnormal motor behaviour*: ways of changing something in desperation, of getting attention for resource access, to provide a distraction, or to avoid future social interactions. These are behaviours that have been shaped under tight social control and the control by language is now weakened.

- *Being reckless, impulsivity*: behaviours shaped by tight social control but the control by language is now weakened, they can also be a form of distraction or to avoid future social interactions.

- *Increased energy*: behaviour shaped by having too many audiences with contradictory demands and the effects and socializing of the capitalist and neoliberal systems, a way of getting attention for resource access, or to avoid future social interactions.

- *Increased spending*: as above but more specific, also to provide a distraction.

- *Overactivity*: as above. Behaviours shaped under tight social control and the control by language is now weakened.

- *Repetitive behaviours applied rigidly*: as above but when shaped in a limited part of life, by the effects and socializing of the capitalist and neoliberal systems to be productive, also as a form of distraction.

(I will come back to this point at the very end, because we will see other examples of there being *similar responses to bad situations* with the only real difference being that some are verbal, some 'emotional' [non-language], and some physical.)

5. Thinking and talking problematic: general

Language issues take up a large part of the DSM, even though they are only talked about abstractly as 'internal cognitive processing' or 'thought disorders'. Ironically, they actually arise from social relationship problems as we saw earlier in this chapter (and V4). Most of our world contexts are about doing things with people to get what we need (and needing reciprocation of course), and the major way we do things with people is through using language, either spoken or through enforced rules (if we have a resource–power differential that we can apply). This means that if one's social relationships and community networks start to fail and are no longer functional or supportive, because of power/social relationship problems, then we will see lots of the 'thinking disorder' or 'cognitive issue' strategies appear in people's behaviours because all their usual language strategies no longer work and they cannot get people to do things anymore. I argue that this change takes place in a changing social world, not inside our head.

This is a very different way of thinking from traditional psychology and everyday talk, so we need to be very clear that issues with language are not about something internal, as psychology promulgates (Pathway 1), but about issues with making things happen (or not happening) through the use of language with other people in that person's world, whether this be 'attributional biases', 'fixed ideas', delusional talk, dysfunctional core beliefs, or 'word salad' (see V4.7 and Chapter 6, Box 6.1). Certain ways of talking have been shaped by the person's social world and these conversational snippets are now causing problems (Pathway 2). When social relationships break down, words no longer function.

> Accordingly, for [the "schizophrenic"], the word is the same as an object [that is, has lost the social functioning], and by analysing the word one learns something about the object [ironically, this is how Western philosophy treats the word]. One of my patients, asked what the acting principle of the world is, answered with "the words". "One can improve one's existence by words. One can influence buying and selling, and one can ruin people by the word 'haha'. Sometimes two or three words are so powerful that one can devitalize several people. There are strong and weak words. One can also take out the words and provoke misfortune and disease. There

are also daring and hearty words. One can find out by them who has done a certain thing."

(Schilder, 1976, p. 317)

This patient has lost the social functioning of words but clearly sees that words are powerful in human life to get anything done. Without the social functioning, *the words can also be used in any way and with any grammar* in attempts to change the state of their social world. My only correction to Schilder is that the words *themselves* are not influential, daring, hearty, ruining, or devitalizing—they are just empty marks on paper or vocal sounds; it is the social relationships and their resource outcomes and reciprocity that make these outcomes happen from these words.

In another way, the more general thought disorders can sometimes be similar in function to the general behaviours, mood changes, and unusual actions seen earlier—they are trying *any* sort of response to change a bad situation because there is either no identified proper response that will change the bad situation, the most useful behaviours are blocked, or else previous attempts have failed. But in the present group, they are trying new *language responses to change social relationships*, rather than being reckless, crying, violent, moody, or overactive. Basically, *the 'overdramatic', erratic, and reckless behaviours equate functionally to 'word salad', as do the general mood changes.*

These behaviours have been grouped together therefore because they apply across a large portion of the person's lifeworlds. They are *general properties of language use* that have been shaped and would usually indicate that an early but important audience was involved in the shaping, or there was shaping over a longer period of time. Most likely there have not been other audiences present to extinguish these behaviours or shape alternatives. But remember that if they become punished socially, they are also likely to become thinking problems rather than problems of talking out loud (V4.4) (see Box 4.4).

Group 2: social behaviours

The next grouping of DSM 'behaviours' were grouped together because they all relate to problematic social relationships, although we must remember that getting and distributing resources will also be at the heart of these problems. As would be expected, most of these are language-based (our main way of working with people) even when not specifically about language per se (e.g. argumentativeness). Similar overlap will occur for behaviours in the fourth grouping, which are directly about language uses.

Box 4.4 The DSM behaviours corresponding to my grouping

Thinking and talking problematic: general (placed into seven groups that seem allied)

1. *Slowing down of thoughts and actions*: if there is a punishing, highly critical social environment (audiences) then there will be a lot of conversation not said out loud (thoughts) and heavily edited, hence slowing might be expected.

   • *Concentration difficulties*: when there are abstract or societal issues shaping the bad situation, the general contexts apply 24/7 so this can affect concentration and lead to being distracted 'for no reason'.

   • *Consciousness disrupted from normal*: when social relationships are disrupted, the corresponding language and thought patterns will also change. In extreme conditions (bad situations) this can lead to unconnected discourses appearing and the sense of regular 'me' thinking disrupted.

   • *Memory disrupted from normal*: memory is language (V4.9) and therefore socially shaped and patterned. When the social lifeworlds get messed up, the normal patterns of remembering will follow suit.

   • *Perception disrupted from normal*: likewise, as for memory above, patterns of observation and patterns of attention are socially controlled to a major degree (V4.5). Much of 'perception' is about socially naming, and this can also be disrupted when social relationships are part of a bad situation.

2. *Racing thoughts*: potentially these are social 'bullying' strategies that have been shaped, talking and thinking rapidly to avoid outcomes from the talk, such as interruptions and criticism.

   • *Rapid speech*: potentially this is a social 'bullying' strategy that has been shaped, talking and thinking rapidly to avoid outcomes from the talk, such as interruptions and criticism.

3. *Disorganized thinking*: following (1) above, the extreme cases with exaggeration will lead to the sorts of experiences captured in these words.

- *Cognitive or perceptual distortions*: following (1) above, the extreme cases with exaggeration will lead to the sorts of experiences captured in these words.
- *Preoccupation*: following (1) above, the extreme cases with exaggeration will lead to the sorts of experiences captured in these words.

4. *Intolerance of uncertainty*: possibly similar to (2) above, to avoid outcomes from the talk, such as interruptions and criticism, distraction.

- *Repetitive mental acts applied rigidly*: distraction possibly, shaped as 'editing' language uses because of punishing or highly critical situations.

There are not many 'symptoms' directly related to social relationships in the DSM, and I believe that this is for a few reasons. First, many 'social relationship' problems get solved before the responses get highly exaggerated, become chronic, and get viewed as 'mental health' disorders; that is, they are social relationship problems not part of any 'bad life situation'. Many are now due to the huge increase in stranger social relationships in modernity, which we have less experience dealing with, but for which we have human resources, police, lawyers, mediators, etc. there to help. Family and spousal social relationships are more about discourses and mismatches of discourses (the resource–social relationship links are the problem, not the words themselves) between people, and counsellors, therapists, and others that are there to help with these. The exceptions are when some of those involved have kept the issues private or secret (as part of the shaped strategizing) and so the issues get worse and no one is there to help solve them (the strategy of social isolation in domestic violence, for example).

Second, we can usually *see* the various people who are in social relationship conflicts so the typically 'hidden' criteria of calling something a 'mental health' problem is not there. People might call their neighbour 'insane' because of what they are doing, but professionals will take both views into account in solving such problems. So, the criteria that 'mental health' issues have hidden sources is usually not there.

Third, many of the social problems become language-use problems that, for traditional psychologists, become seen as individual 'cognitive' problems and the social dimension is lost (V5.1). We will deal with these cases in the third grouping of DSM symptoms and bring the 'social' back in again. These social problems are wrongly treated as individual 'thinking' or 'cognition' problems with the social contexts excluded, when in fact the social problems in the bad situations are the most important (cf. V5.1).

Some of these, however, will have developed into chronic social relationship problems, and be exaggerated and become trapped over time by the context (such as domestic violence situations). Others will arise from life issues perhaps not directly about social relationships, but they are again some sort of response to try and change bad situations through changing the social relationships. It might be difficult to distinguish these, but check who is supporting these behaviours (that is, who listens to them, responds in any way to them, is involved in the life situation, does the person only refer to abstract or stranger effects, etc.).

Fourth, the fewer social relationship problems than might be expected is also an artefact, however, of dividing (forcing) human life into mental versus non-mental health problems (see Chapter 8 and V4). Most of the 'social relationship' problems get dealt with by other professionals and do not make it to the DSM. As outlined above, this is not because they are not serious problems but because the environmental functioning is more salient. The ones that make it to the DSM are merely those that have become locked in, entrenched, or chronic, and those for which the contexts are difficult to see so they are then treated wrongly as intractable internal issues originating inside the person. But I have urged, as many now have, that this mental/non-mental distinction is an artefact of how much time we spend engaging with people and looking for the contextual problems.

The final reason why social relationship problems are sparse in the DSM is that problems with language use conceal social relationship problems. What are seen as 'functional speech disorders' and 'functional thought disorders' are really problems with social relationships, and for the latter saying things to change the situation out loud has been punished by social relationships so they become thoughts (V4.4). And there are lots of them! We will see this in what follows and *they could have been placed in this section if the social basis of language use and thinking were better understood by clinicians.*

4. Social relationships problematic

The behaviours that are listed in the DSM involving social relationships are mostly still viewed as the 'individual' pathology of one of the people in the relationship, especially if the influence of the other people is hidden. Unless you believe in spontaneous brain diseases, there is always more going on in the social contexts if you know how to observe and contextualize properly (see Box 4.5).

Box 4.5 The DSM behaviours corresponding to my grouping

Social relationships problematic (placed into seven groups that seem allied)

- *Detachment from social relationships, lack of empathy, social inhibition*: possible historical or contemporary contexts of people or society punishing both social behaviours and uses of language. The person is foregoing resources or has alternative ways of getting resources that do not require social relationships (prevalent under capitalism). Human resources come through resource–social relationship pathways so the person has a way of surviving this. Under capitalism all resources and relationships can be done with money and strangers, so money is the key.

- *Disregard for the rights of others*: similar to the above.

- *Acute discomfort in close relationships, interpersonal relationships instability*: history of resource–social relationship pathways going wrong, difficulties with stranger exchanges or contractual relationships in the modern world.

- *Submissive and clinging behaviour*: avoidance of other relationships, especially dealing with modern stranger social relationships and their vagaries, behaviour is shaped to remain in current social relationships at all costs.

- *Argumentativeness, defiance, opposition behaviour*: rightly or wrongly the person does not wish to change their resource–social relationship pathways. Behaviour may be shaped by hidden resource access the other person cannot see, avoidance of alternative events that the other person cannot see, or beliefs tied in with specific and powerful resource–social relationship pathways and holding on to beliefs for these is more important than the immediate effects of argumentativeness or irritability. May also be a strategy of bullying that might be irrelevant to what is being argued about or what is being opposed, or part of another strategy.

- *Irritability, intermittent explosive irritation, intermittent explosive anger, intermittent explosive behaviours*: escalations or exaggerations of the above.

- *Self-control problems that bring significant conflict, emotional self-control problems that bring significant conflict*: self-control is shaped socially (V5.5) so there are again problems with the person's social relationships (not their brain) and these either use words in the first case or words are not working in the second case so 'emotional' responses occur.

5. *Thinking and talking problematic: talking about social relationships*

While all talking is shaped by social relationships, these are behaviours that are specifically about the relationships themselves and go beyond 'mere' interpersonal problems. 'Self-control' problems could be included here if the link was understood better (V4.4, V5.6) (see Box 4.6).

Group 3: language and discourse issues

Thinking and talking: introduction

Language issues take up a large part of the DSM, even though they are talked about as individualistic 'internal cognitive processing', 'mental' problems, or 'thought disorders' (Pathway 1). Ironically, they are really social relationship problems as was described earlier in this chapter (and V4). Most of our world contexts are about doing things with people to get what we need (unless you are totally self-sufficient), and the major way we do things with people is through using language, either spoken or through enforced rules. This means that if one's use of language starts to fail and is no longer functional, because of bad social situations or power/social relationship problems, then we will see lots of the 'thinking disorders' or 'cognitive issues' strategies shaped in people's behaviours to change this. But I argue (V4.8) that this is because the social reciprocity resource exchanges are faulty (Pathway 2), not because of 'faulty' language or thinking (Pathway 1).

Box 4.6 The DSM behaviours corresponding to my grouping

Thinking and talking problematic: talking about social relationships (placed into two groups that seem allied)

- *Distrust and suspiciousness of others' motives*: many external contexts could produce this, prior punishment, tenuous resource–social relationship pathways, too many short stranger-based exchanges and social relationships.
- *Need for admiration*: while possibly related to the earlier contextualized 'attachment', it can form part of many other strategies arising from diverse contexts.

So, we need to be very clear that issues with language are not about something internal, but about making things happen (or not) in the person's *social world* through the use of language with people, whether this be 'attributional biases', 'fixed ideas', delusional talk, identity issues, dysfunctional core beliefs, or word salad (see earlier in this chapter, Chapter 6, V5.5, and V4.8). Certain ways of talking have been shaped by the person's social world and these conversational snippets are now causing problems.

Finally, we saw that thinking is just talking but not out loud (V4.4) so if the talking out loud is punished or the person has been silenced socially or societally, then we are more likely to find 'thought disorder' diagnoses (Table 4.1 in V4). Ironically, most people see these as the quintessential *private behaviours* in the head, but they are really external social behaviours and indicate that social relationships and social exchanges have gone sour, and especially when trying to talk out loud to change what people are doing and therefore change the bad situations.

6. Thinking and talking problematic: specific

These behaviours have been put together merely because they are specific to audiences, contexts, or situations and they do not figure in the remaining three groups. While unwanted or intrusive thoughts are common in both everyday and 'dysfunctional' forms, they include certain specific forms that need attention in contextual analysis. In each case we must remember that these are shaped behaviours, but only shaped by people, and they can be shaped by avoidance as well as by leading to the things we need in life.

These are all functionally identical to the 'actions unusual' category given earlier but they involve or utilize language instead of more physical or 'emotional' responses (like overly dramatic gestures or moods; this will be summarized at the end of this chapter). Once again, we need to remember that these arise in our social and discursive worlds, not inside the head. Language only has consequences by affecting people, so we must ask the question: what sorts of context does this person live in that these ways of talking (and therefore thinking) were shaped by other people or at least not discouraged early on before getting exaggerated and chronic? And like the earlier category of 'actions unusual', we must ask why they are using and then exaggerating language responses to try and get what they want in their worlds (see Box 4.7).

Box 4.7 The DSM behaviours corresponding to my grouping

Thinking and talking problematic: specific

- *Delusions*: behaviour shaped to get social attention to develop resource–social relationship pathways originally. Abstract stories are difficult for people to challenge (even therapists report this) so they can be upheld. They can provide discourses for the person in all parts of life, although this can be more difficult as they get exaggerated, and they provide stories that can be given for social interactions, although again this gets more difficult as they get exaggerated. They can also provide distractions.
- *Dysfunctional beliefs*: mostly as above and analysed in V4.7, variations of argumentativeness, defiance, and opposition behaviours seen earlier. As strategies, the content might not be all that relevant to the bad situation and should not be over-interpreted. They might be the only 'attention-getting' stories they have.
- *Intrusive and unwanted thoughts*: all thoughts are intrusive, but the special character of the ones referred to in this way probably related most to the 'unwanted' property—that they provide contradictions between audiences and the person does not 'want' this thought to appear—if the bad situation is powerful then these unwanted thoughts will remain.
- *Grandiose ideas, grandiosity*: exaggerated versions of most of the above. Performs a similar function to being overly dramatic and suggests that the person's normal talking is failing to develop resource–social relationship pathways for them.
- *Hallucinations*: as seen in V4.5, the occurrence of imagery (re-responding in the same way as when directly reacting to the world) is common. We do not use imagery or sensations to 'perceive' but the perceptual responding can be 're-responded' and it then appears as if we are 'perceiving' the objects or scene again. It is also *socially based* in that what we see and mostly what we report are about our social contexts and resource–social relationship pathways. Sometimes this is all verbal and reports of 'seeing' without the objects are more like language use. All this exaggerated would be just like 'seeing' hallucinations but they usually cannot then be 'explored' except verbally, so the experience is real and usually scary because the non-exploration gives what is 'seen' (re-responded') a sense of being unusual—which it is. The reporting of hallucinations, at least under Western conditions, is likely to lead to other symptoms.
- *Recurrent and persistent thoughts*: similar to 'intrusive' and unwanted thoughts but exaggerating.

Some points for analysis coming from Volume 4 are relevant here (V4.4, V4.7):

- We all hear voices and have intrusive thoughts. All our thoughts are intrusive in fact because they are not shaped by 'us' inside but by our *discursive worlds* and they just 'pop into our heads'.
- So one question, then, is: in what life situations are thoughts said to be 'intrusive' or voices gain so much attention for people (Luhrmann et al., 2019)? This is a societal issue.
- We all have *multiple language responses* to almost any situation since talking about things is overlearned, but only one can get said (except for those with 'rapid speech' as well). Indeed, Freud's goal was to get his clients saying as many thoughts as possible out loud.
- As is well known in 'hearing voices' groups, the problem is more about *managing* our multiple language responses (voices) rather than getting rid of them.
- So another question is: if someone begins saying the more weird or disconnected thoughts arising from their life situations, how is it that these are not punished by other people (the person could be isolated, have weak social relationships with strangers only, their social relationships generally are critical ones so the thoughts are strong but never said out loud to be consequated, they could be using 'bullying beliefs' with exaggerated language or gestures and others just seem to go along with them)?
- Another question is: how is it that one thought/voice becomes strong, and in some cases becomes the person's 'me', critical, or 'command' voice? Where have the other voices gone?
- We can all have strange thoughts arising from life situations (sometimes when responding with humour), so how are these normally managed that they do not become problems (are they punished because they are usually tried out loud, do other critical discourses weaken them)?
- Are there major problems because in the bad life situation *most* language is punished (living in very criticizing social relationships) and so most of the person's language is never said out loud and consequated? They end up with more thoughts than spoken words.
- The 'bad' thoughts or voices do not control the person's behaviour (V5.6). But they do provide ways in which 'odd' behaviour can be justified afterwards to other people as excuses, stories, explanations, etc.
- Some might arise from bad situations in which there are mainly criticizing audiences and the 'me' voices (those that justify what the person is doing and saying they will do) never get said out loud, so the

justifications, stories, and excuses become focused on bad or bizarre future events and do not get consequated at that point as might have happened otherwise.

- We must remember that Freud had problems getting people to say out loud more than their usual 'me' thoughts, especially if strong punishment ('repression') had come from the person's contexts.

- We also need to consider the contexts in which the 'intrusive', bizarre, or negative thoughts finally *do* get said out loud, to a therapist or someone else. There is no catharsis (as Freud might say) but the thoughts finally get socially consequated, and only then can provide new possibilities for resource–social relationship pathways in the future, which might allow the current bad situation to change.

- First-hand experiencers of these behaviours often say that one of the important things about recovery was to find some *social connection* with people who are not critical of what they are reporting—even strangers (for example with emotional-CPR methods). Therapists such as within CBT are often focused, however, on *getting rid* of these 'symptoms' as soon as possible, or getting other thoughts to distract. These can have the paradoxical effect of shaping the thoughts to appear more often as thoughts rather than as talking out loud, and occurring more often anyway since they changed the person's world a little.

- But it will probably not help just saying these sorts of thoughts freely out loud ('catharsis') without shaping new ways forward to resources and social relationships with good interdependencies and not criticism. We need to help people *rebuild their concrete, material lives* and not just get rid of the 'symptoms'; just saying them out loud in the wrong contexts could make matters worse. When Freud got the person to say the 'repressed' thought out loud and they were 'cured', he must have done other things to change the person's resource–social relationship pathways on the basis of these thoughts; there was no catharsis leading to a cure (Guerin, 2001)

- As an initial stage it could be useful to get people with these symptoms to say them *out loud* but all by themselves, or, as we will see in Chapter 6, say them out loud to a god, spirit, or an imaginary being (depending upon their other beliefs); later they can be said out loud to a 'safe' person such as a therapist or friend.

7. Thinking and talking problematic: identity talk

To understand the importance of identity talk (V5.5), and why it figures so largely in the DSM, requires going back to the basic properties of language given earlier: *we get all our resources of life through people, and we influence people predominantly through our uses of language.* This means that how we present ourselves to others (in deeds and talk) is vital for our life resources, both in other people attending to us at all, and to how we then build a relationship with exchanges of resources (V5). If you are in a bad and inescapable lifeworld then all these will suffer.

As we saw earlier in this chapter, once upon a time, our families were the main source of relationships leading to resources, but this has hugely changed. To get what we need in life (friendships, jobs, money, entertainment, etc.) we now need to build many relationships with people who are initially strangers, that is, non-kin. One of the properties of non-kin is that they often do not know you very well or have probably only known you for a short period of time. In large extended families, everyone has known everyone for many years, and possibly for their whole life.

What this quick review of social relationships tells us is that the properties of how we present ourselves to others is very different now in modernity (with compartmentalization). We must let many strangers in many different parts of our life know what we are like because they have *not* known us all our lives, but we can also make things up or exaggerate as long as they cannot check easily. So, presenting an identity, which is now primarily about talking or buying things, is now fraught with new problems and requires many strategies.

But again, we must remember (V4.6) that this is not just a matter of words: "Shall I describe myself this way or that way?" Our identities are our means of getting into resource–social relationship pathways and involve actions, although less so in the modern world since we run our lives through money and resources produced and distributed by other people. In modern times, getting resources can depend far more on 'talking the talk' than having to 'walk the walk'. This is probably also why there are now more problems and issues around talking and thinking than just about access to resources, and why 'cognitive' (= language use) approaches are so prevalent in therapies.

For contextualizing identity talk we also have to remember that a functional identity does not always mean a 'good' or 'nice' identity. *A functional identity is one that influences people to get the outcomes we think we want or need, or else it avoids what we do not want or need*, and these can include, for example, being a goth or emo, or criminal activities and bullying (Rowe & Guerin, 2018). We get pathways to live, whether these are viewed as good or bad by others.

Like all these categories of DSM 'symptoms', all of those listed in Box 4.8 from the DSM are behaviours seen in everyday life and *the approach should really be about locating the bad life situations that have shaped these normal behaviours to become exaggerated, and made them*

Box 4.8 The DSM behaviours corresponding to my grouping

Thinking and talking problematic: identity talk (placed into five groups that seem allied)

- *Identity disrupted from normal, self-image instability*: as self-identity depends upon the external (mainly social) contexts, this merely indicates that things are bad in the person's situation, or changing. If the bad situation is changing quickly then there will be instability, if the bad situation is shaping two or more identities that are contradictory in some ways, then this is how the person's identity/identities will appear. If the audiences for each identity can be kept separate then there might be no issues. The 'need' to be consistent also needs contextualizing (Guerin, 2016) since it is not always necessary and is itself a social demand.

- *Hypersensitivity to negative evaluation, finding it hard to take minor personal criticisms, feelings of inadequacy*: all these are normal but have been exaggerated in a bad situation. As they have become more general (not just negative evaluation on one activity) then it is likely that the bad situation in this person's life is arising from societal contexts or highly interdependent social relationships (doing badly in one activity will be reflected on all the others). These behaviours have possible shaping from the generic capitalist and neoliberal worlds we live in.

- *Need to control thoughts, perfectionism preoccupation, orderliness preoccupation, inflated sense of responsibility*: similar to the above.

- *Suicide thoughts*: possible escaping from bad situations totally without promise of fitting into life through any resource–social relationship pathways, or possible action to prevent making those in social relationships from having bad situations because of your behaviour that you do not understand either. These are exaggerated normal thoughts of escape or avoidance, which means that the person's environment is bad and needs changing. The thoughts are not instructions that will be followed, since this is a false idea of everyday thoughts (V4; V5.5).

- *Body representation disrupted from normal, increased physical health complaints, disturbance of thoughts and talk about eating, or eating-related behaviour*: when language strategies and moods are not effective in changing the bad situations in life, these are always possible as attempts to change things since food and eating will be ongoing and social events. Complaining and discourses of body 'representations' are a verbal form.

locked in to become chronic, rather than look for the origin of the behaviour inside the person or making interpretations of the specific behaviours.

The worlds we live in shape our attempted identities. So, all these behaviours are about problems with a bad life situation (or else they would be solved simply and quickly) and issues with people (possibly abstract discursive others) in trying to plan or carry out forms of resource–social relationship pathways to get by in life.

9. Thinking and talking problematic: anxiety and fear

These are a well-known set of behaviours although they are still very complex for analysis. Some, like phobias, might not always seem to be language-based, but the person is still reacting quickly and strongly to words.

All are based on being shaped into *abstract discourses of problems with resource–social relationship pathways* that are normal but exaggerated and persistent in bad situations. Generalized anxiety is abstract and possibly due to *societal* shaping of the bad situations (which means that little can be done as actions to change this Chapters 7 and 8). Talking out loud does not always help despite supportive social relationships, or is punished, so thinking results.

As before, the topography or verbal content of the anxiety might not be important and should not always be over-interpreted, although it might give clues to the bad life situation. But if the person does not know the abstract, societal contexts from which the bad situations arise then the anxiety content could be irrelevant. In either case the behaviours need contextualizing to the bad situation and work done on changing those, rather than just trying to stop or distract (CBT) the anxiety talk (see Box 4.9).

Box 4.9 The DSM behaviours corresponding to my grouping

Thinking and talking problematic: anxiety and fear (placed into three groups that seem allied)

- *Nervousness, worry, generalized anxiety, anxiety, appear anxious or fearful, excessive fear and anxiety, agoraphobia, panic attacks*: bad situations and attempts to change are not working, talking out loud about concerns can then be punished into thinking patterns instead. Features of the earlier 'general behaviours' category above also appear. Contextualizing to locate the bad situations is probably more useful than arguing over the anxiety content.

- *Phobias*: just more specific versions of the above usually, but this can also potentially have a phobia that is irrelevant. The person strategically appears more in control if just a single object phobia than if their whole world is falling apart. If desensitization does not work then the latter might be checked.
- *Overestimating threat*: similar patterns but language-based so used socially as explanations, justifications, conversational stories, etc.

Summary

As mentioned at the start, all of the points raised in this chapter are not meant as any sort of final or definitive proof. The aim was not *factual* but *practical*—to alter the reader's way of observing people and analysing what they do to transform from (Pathway 1) to (Pathway 2). The only way ahead is to examine real cases and switch the focus from 'getting a disorder label' to finding the bad contexts that shaped these 'mental health' behaviours and work to change those bad situations for the person.

Functional links needed

What links all these 'symptoms' is not a common brain disorder but common *situational conditions*. I have tried to shape the reader away from the DSM groupings and into more functional groupings based on context. Much more of this needs to be done, but if this thinking can help break the pattern of observing and analysing, then the aim has been reached.

To finish, Table 4.1 presents a summary of one of the suggestions made incidentally above; that some of the symptom groups seem to be functionally equivalent even though the DSM places them as very distinct 'disorders'.

What this suggests is that someone can be shaped to escape or change their bad situation, and if they have spent their life doing things to people with words this could be shaped in the extreme into delusions, grandiose ideas, or hallucinations. If they have not used words heavily in their life to solve problems, they might have been shaped to use more physical actions and in extreme cases develop symptoms of recklessness, overactivity, or odd physical behaviours. In the absence of both physical or verbal ways to change their bad situation, they might be shaped into non-language-based actions of moodiness, hopelessness, or affective instability.

Table 4.1 Three groups of very different-looking behaviours that might have been shaped in the same functional way but have emerged differently because the background life shaping has focused on physical, emotional, or verbal strategies for the person

Background	Strategies that have been shaped	Behaviour
When the person has been socialized to be more physical than verbal (need to find out the contexts that produced this), or in social relationships with people not excessively verbal so words do not work anyway	Mostly physical	Appear dramatic, emotional, or erratic Appear odd or eccentric, eccentricities of behaviour Disorganized or abnormal motor behaviour Being reckless, impulsivity Increased energy Increased spending Overactivity Repetitive behaviours applied rigidly
Person has been in bad situations with real social relationships for which words were not functioning well, perhaps because the environment is full of critical or toxic people or relationships are failing (people not reciprocating to requests or people not listening)	Mostly 'emotional' (non-language)	Affective instability Emotion disrupted from normal Empty mood Excessive emotionality Hopelessness Moodiness that is out of character Lack of enjoyment, loss of interest in pleasurable activities Restricted range of emotional expression Sad mood, sadness
Bad situations that are abstract, in the past, involve stranger relationships, or arise from societal 'structures'; when the person has been taught to rely on words when things need changing but that is not working perhaps because they have no close social relationships to help anyway, or else 'normal' talking for persuasion gets nowhere	Mostly discursive	Delusions Dysfunctional beliefs Intrusive and unwanted thoughts Grandiose ideas, grandiosity Hallucinations Recurrent and persistent thoughts

References

Barker, R., Dembo, T., & Lewin, K. (1941/1976). *Frustration and regression: An experiment with young children.* New York, NY: Arno Press.

Bleuler, E. (1911/1950). *Dementia praecox or the group of schizophrenias.* New York, NY: International Universities Press.

Bleuler, E. (1912). *The theory of schizophrenic negativism.* New York, NY: Johnson Reprint.

Broug, M. (2008). *Seventeen voices: Life and wisdom from inside 'mental illness'.* Adelaide: Wakefield Press.

Cameron, N., & Magaret, A. (1951). *Behavior pathology.* Boston, MA: Houghton Mifflin.

Campbell, C. M. (1925). *A present-day conception of mental disorders.* Cambridge, MA: Harvard University Press.

Cleckley, H. (1964). *The mask of sanity: An attempt to clarify some issues about the so-called psychopathic personality.* Saint Louis, MI: C. V. Mosby.

Costello, C. G. (Ed.) (1970). *Symptoms of psychopathology: A handbook.* New York, NY: John Wiley.

de Rivera, J. (1976). *Field theory as human-science: Contributions of Lewin's Berlin group.* New York, NY: Gardner Press.

Dorman, P. (2006). *I cry for help: Autobiography/health, my true story detailing the aftermath of child abuse, trauma, stress, combat trauma, and post-traumatic stress disorder.* New York, NY: iUniverse.

#Emerging Proud. (2019). *Through trauma and abuse: Stories of hope & transformation.* Norwich, UK: Emerging Proud Press.

Factora-Borchers, L. (Ed.) (2014). *Dear sister: Letters from survivors of sexual abuse.* Edinburgh: AK Press.

Fromene, R., & Guerin, B. (2014). Talking to Australian Indigenous clients with borderline personality disorder labels: Finding the context behind the diagnosis. *Psychological Record, 64*, 569–579.

Fromene, R., Guerin, B., & Krieg, A. (2014). Australian Indigenous clients with a borderline personality disorder diagnosis: A contextual review of the literature. *Psychological Record, 64*, 559–567.

Guerin, B. (1992). Social behavior as discriminative stimulus and consequence in social anthropology. *Behavior Analyst, 15*, 31–41.

Guerin, B. (2001). Replacing catharsis and uncertainty reduction theories with descriptions of the historical and social context. *Review of General Psychology, 5*, 44–61.

Guerin, B. (2005). *Handbook of interventions for changing people and communities.* Reno, NV: Context Press.

Guerin, B. (2016). *How to rethink human behavior: A practical guide to social contextual analysis.* London: Routledge.

Guerin, B. (2017). *How to rethink mental illness: The human contexts behind the labels.* London: Routledge.

Guerin, B. (2018). The use of participatory and non-experimental research methods in behavior analysis. *Revista Perspectivas em Análise Comportamento, 9*, 248–264.

Guerin, B. (2019). What do therapists and clients talk about when they cannot explain behaviours? How Carl Jung avoided analysing a client's environments by inventing theories. *Revista Perspectivas em Análise Comportamento, 10*, 76–97.

Guerin, B., & Guerin, P. (2012). Re-thinking mental health for indigenous Australian communities: Communities as context for mental health. *Community Development Journal, 47*(4), 555–570.

Guerin, B., Leugi, G. B., & Thain, A. (2018). Attempting to overcome problems shared by both qualitative and quantitative methodologies: Two hybrid procedures to encourage diverse research. *Australian Community Psychologist, 29*, 74–90.

Janet, P. (1902). *The mental state of hystericals: A study of mental stigmata and mental accidents.* New York, NY: G. P. Putnam's Sons.

Janet, P. (1907). *The major symptoms of hysteria.* London: Macmillan.

Johnstone, L., Boyle, M., Cromby, J., Dillon, J., Harper, D., Kinderman, P., … Read, J. (2018). *The Power Threat Meaning Framework: Towards the identification of patterns in emotional distress, unusual experiences and troubled or troubling behaviour, as an alternative to functional psychiatric diagnosis.* Leicester, UK: British Psychological Society.

Jung, C. G., (1960). *The psychogenesis of mental disease.* New York, NY: Princeton University Press.

Longden, E., Corstens, D., Escher, S., & Romme, M. (2012). Voice hearing in a biographical context: A model for formulating the relationship between voices and life history. *Psychosis, 4*, 224–234.

Luhrmann, T. M., Alderson-Day, B., Bell, V., Bless, J. J., Corlett, P., Hugdahl, K. … Waters, F. (2019). Beyond trauma: A multiple pathways approach to auditory hallucinations in clinical and non-clinical populations. *Schizophrenia Bulletin, 45*, S24–S31.

Meyer, A. (1948). *The commonsense psychiatry of Dr. Alfred Meyer: Fifty-two selected papers, with biographical narrative.* New York, NY: McGraw-Hill.

Mills, C. W. (1959). *The sociological imagination.* Oxford: Oxford University Press.

Rogers, K. L., & Leydesdorff, S. (2004). *Trauma: Life stories of survivors.* London: Transaction Publishers.

Romme, M., Escher, S., Dillon, J., Corstens, D., & Morris, M. (2009). *Living with voices: 50 stories of recovery.* London: PCCS Books.

Rowe, P. (2018). *Heavy metal youth identities: Researching the musical empowerment of youth transitions and psychosocial wellbeing.* London: Emerald Publishing.

Rowe, P., & Guerin, B. (2018). Contextualizing the mental health of metal youth: A community for social protection, identity and musical empowerment. *Journal of Community Psychology, 46*, 1–13.

Ryan, J., Guerin, P., Elmi, F. H., & Guerin, B. (2019). What can Somali community talk about mental health tell us about our own? Contextualizing the symptoms of mental health. *International Journal of Migration, Health and Social Care, 15*, 13–24.

Schilder, P. (1950). *The image and the appearance of the human body: Studies in the constructive energies of the psyche.* New York, NY: International Universities Press.

Schilder, P. (1976). *On psychoses.* New York, NY: International Universities Press.

Schneider, B. (2010). *Hearing (our) voices: Participatory research in mental health.* Toronto, ON: University of Toronto Press.

Sears, R. R. (1941). II. Non-aggressive reactions to frustration. *Psychological Review, 48,* 343–346.

Sullivan, H. S. (1973). *Clinical studies in psychiatry.* New York, NY: Norton.

Sullivan, H. S. (1974). *Schizophrenia as a human process.* New York, NY: Norton.

Watson, J. (2019). *Drop the disorder: Challenging the culture of psychiatric diagnosis.* London: PCCS Books.

Wyatt-Brown, B. (1988). The mask of obedience: Male slave psychology in the old South. *American Historical Review, 93,* 1228–1252.

Xinran (2002). *The good women of China: Hidden voices.* London: Vintage Books.

5 How can we change behaviour by changing local bad situations?

> I know! It is pretty bloody clear I needed to just concentrate on fixing my situation from the beginning—all this awful dance has done has taken my attention away from that. I've completely put my life on the back burner to try and pay attention to my head and the result is a shitstorm that gets worse every day. I'm so scared of this journey.
>
> (Anonymous first-hand experiencer, personal communication)

Currently, 'mental health' professionals' energy is focused on fitting very abstract and generic groups of 'symptoms' into abstract categories of 'disorders'. For example, "The client shows 'disordered thinking' and therefore seems to *have* a psychosis" (Pathway 1). This approach needs to stop as I believe it is extremely superficial, even apart from the DSM classification having innumerable problems (Watson, 2019). The 'individual behaviours' are put into abstract categories of 'symptoms', and these abstract categories are then put into *even more abstract* categories of 'disorders'. Further, and unlike general medical practice, the disorders do not have specific and reliable 'treatments' of what to do next. *Diagnoses are currently an end point* rather than signalling an associated form of treatment, as happens in general medical practice.

This DSM focus on categorization has also *distracted* professionals from observing more specific details of people and their contexts. The focus is on observing or asking the client just enough to make a diagnosis, and all context is then lost. If they report anxious thinking, then that is enough to know because a diagnosis can be given. With the major changes suggested here in the thinking about psychology (V1, V2, V4), we now need a new focus (Pathway 2), which broadly will be along these lines (see also Johnstone et al., 2018; Schwarz & Goldiamond, 1975; Watson, 2019):

- What has happened to you? What bad situations were you in or are you in?

- If the bad situation is current, how can we change your life contexts *to relieve this first of all*, and then *to change your bad situation*?
- If the bad situation was some time ago, what happened to your other life contexts back then that still leaves you in a bad situation, and how can we change these?
- What *specific* actions, talk, or thinking have been shaped in these bad situations?
- What needs changing in your world?
- Can you put into words what the bad situations are and what they are shaping you to do?
- Will you allow me to go into your world and observe your total contexts?
- What resources do you have and what do you need? To achieve these, what social relationships do you have and what do you need?
- What did those specific behaviours originally attempt to change do you think? Have they worked?
- What would life be like if you stopped these behaviours?

The key thing is to put the main *observational and analytic focus on the person's bad contexts*, which are shaping the behaviours that are giving them problems. *Interventions should be focused on how to change those bad situations* for this person. My vision for the future would be losing the titles of our current 'experts' (psychology, psychiatry, social work, counselling) and developing people who are *experts in certain types of bad situations* and how to fix them, or how to relieve the people caught in them if they cannot be fixed easily. This would include those with first-hand experience and those who have experience in bad situations that produce behaviours other than just the current 'mental health' behaviours (see Chapter 3).

Changing environments to change behaviour

The following are suggestions about how to try new ways to intervene with people and help them. I certainly do not pretend that these are the final word, and the purpose is really to give at least one new approach to start the changes to 'mental health' interventions. The whole thinking around 'mental health' treatment needs shaking up and being detached from the complacency born of the DSM, faulty cognitive processing, brain malfunction 'explanations', and other assorted medical approaches to 'mental health'.

Currently, I believe, any new approach would help, so here is one to stir things up (see also Johnstone et al., 2018; Watson, 2019). It is more a framework within which practitioners can develop their own approaches based on observing contextually the behaviours and bad situations of each client. For example, the contextual answer to "How should I help this person who is hearing voices?" is always, "It depends'. But from all the six volumes in this series and the guiding framework here, along with the writers and practitioners I have integrated and referenced, we can discover new ways to intervene. The key thing is that the observations and analyses need to be grounded in each client's real-life bad contexts.

From the viewpoint of social contextual analysis then, the simple catch-phrase for intervention or change is: *if someone wants to change their actions, talking, or thinking, they must change those parts of their environments that are shaping and maintaining them.* Easy! However, as we have seen, there are two important and overarching problems:

- identifying the environments that shape the behaviours, especially for the 'mental health' behaviours where they are (by my definition) not easily observable (especially talking, thinking, and bad situations created by societal pressures);
- finding ways to change the impact of societal and discursive systems if they are shaping a person's behaviour, talking, and thinking.

These 'problems' are also the reason why psychotherapists have not taken this route (see Chapter 1). Those trying this same catchphrase ("Change behaviour by changing the environment") for interventions in the 1960s and 1970s under rubrics of 'behaviour therapy' or 'behaviour modification', took only the simplest ideas of 'behaviour being shaped by the environment'. The behaviour modification approaches were reasonably good (1) for simply shaped behaviours, which were easily observable, (2) for overlaying artificial shaping to simply increase or decrease behaviours, and (3) for people with limited or rigid repertoires of behaviours.

But while what they did was of value for some issues, they did not have the analyses or thinking for all the complexity of social, cultural, and societal influences, which of course are also what shape the most complex 'mental health' problems. And like most psychologists and psychiatrists, they had no training for a 'sociological imagination' (Mills, 1959). Those who were dealing with issues around talking or thinking, *really* could not see how these behaviours could be shaped by environments (hence cognitive and brain theories and metaphors were brought in and we ended up with totally abstract cognitive behaviour therapy models). They still 'invented' some CBT techniques that have been effective, but these have been known for a long time in history (Janet, 1919/1925), such as many are new names for Buddhist and Greek techniques that have been used for centuries.

What social contextual analysis tries to add are (1) the ways in which the social systemic environments shape many problematic behaviours and thoughts, and (2) the more concrete grounding of language use and thinking into social audiences and discursive communities. And with these two tools we can at least map out what needs to be done to change bad situations and hence behaviours, even if that task is a big one and not always achievable by individuals (see Chapters 7 and 8).

But thinking in this way also allows us to rethink how we might intervene and change more local issues as well. Local issues with social relationships and money problems are common (because money is our major access to resources in life now). While we do not have to analyse big societal structures into every one of these problems, it is wise to keep in mind that the people or groups on both sides of local conflicts will still be shaped within these big systems, usually by stratification of opportunities, so a sociological imagination is needed even with 'local' issues (as social workers know).

I will divide all the problems and issues into eight topics spread over the following four chapters as follows, although this division is for pedagogy and for breaking up the complacent ways of thinking about therapy currently:

1. Trying to prevent local resource and social relationship issues becoming bad situations.
2. Life problems with observable local resource and social relationship issues.
3. Bad life problems involving 'thinking'.
4. Bad life problems with hidden bad situations but not considered 'mental health' issues.
5. Bad life problems with hidden bad situations and considered 'mental health' issues.
6. Bad life problems with hidden bad societal situations.
7. Indigenous approaches: working with colonization and its aftermath.
8. Feminist approaches: working with the bad situations of women in society.

The main division is between 'local' issues of conflict over resources and social relationships (this chapter), and societal shaping of more hidden issues (see Chapters 7 and 8). I will also separate interventions for talking and thinking, however, since there are so many unique aspects to these and so many previous pitfalls in analysis (see Chapter 6).

Local issues of resources and social relationships

The local issues can be dealt with by many people known to those involved or by many sorts of professionals, and do not usually need specialists. In Western societies, these people can be family and friends, counsellors, church leaders, social workers, imam, financial advisors, online counsellors, etc. In kin-based groups living 'traditionally', the communities often had oral histories of ways to solve such problems, and a range of elders, healers, and religious leaders could help (Gluckman, 1965, 1972; Roberts, 1979).

Trying to prevent local resource and social relationship issues becoming bad situations in the first place

Before looking at interventions for resources and social relationships, there is an important topic to be covered briefly first. This is the problem of not recognizing that people are in bad situations until it is too late. This is especially a problem in Western societies because we increasingly tend to deal mostly with people who are strangers and who have no obligation to us, and we have much less monitoring done by family and friends, so getting into early bad situations might not be seen by anyone at all (and for strangers it is "not my problem"). To exacerbate these problems, the individualistic legal framework means that going for help because of bad situations in life is considered private and confidential, so telling issues to, say, a counsellor, means that the counsellor is not allowed to involve your family and friends (who are probably in the same bad situation) without your permission. Families might not even know that a member has got to the point of seeking help. It is not that people now are any worse, but, I argue, that our *life situations* are worse.

There are some interventions that seek to predict which individuals are likely to develop 'mental illnesses' and do something to prevent this (sometimes called 'prodromal', to mimic medical models). Since these are viewed as internal brain developments that will predict outcomes, drugs medications are usually the outcomes given to young people for prevention. Clearly, the idea itself is a good one, but not the procedure of assessing an 'individual' for signs of 'deteriorating brain issues' and then giving them drugs.

Instead, we need to focus on *early bad situations* and *early life situations that are becoming bad*—'prodromal bad situations', in other words. This already occurs in most kin-based communities because (1) there is a lot of monitoring of people; (2) there are many known people who can intervene and help, and are even *obligated* to help (without requiring money); (3) bad situations (at least pre-colonization) arose from within community relations and so the bigger problems would be known already; and (4) there would be a long oral history of common bad community situations and how to deal with them (e.g. traditional healers, Koran readings, dances and trances, elders, religious rites, community meetings, community parties, etc.).

In Western modernity, however, because of the changes in both resources and social relationships (V5.3), we have bad situations that can continue and no one knows about them before the person becomes trapped into a chronic bad situation, or no one is in a legal position to intervene and support the people involved even if they did know about it. There are too many cases of abuse in childhood in which people (adults) knew what was happening and did nothing, either because they could not legally do anything, or because they did not know how to do this (messed-up social relationships).

Once again, because I am no longer wanting to separate those bad situation outcomes called 'mental health' and those called violence, deception, exploitation, cheating, criminal, etc., all people including professionals who are involved in dealing with any of these outcome behaviours of bad situations could pool ideas and resources if our aim was less about the person and more about the bad situations developing in their lives.

Life problems with observable local resource and social relationship issues

There are innumerable ways to solve local conflicts that are usually about resources, social relationships, or linking these into resource–social relationship pathways, and most carers, counsellors, social workers, clinical psychologists, have skills for this. Usually this requires ways of:

- fixing resources for the person;
- fixing social relationships (need to know social properties of different relationships);
- using social connections to build resource–social relationship pathways;
- distracting from the problems if necessary.

Table 5.1 presents, in an abstract form (cf. Chapter 3), the main resource–social relationship problems with some abstract ideas to solve them.

There are many people who can help with these changes: family, friends, church members, elders, community leaders, social workers, psychologists, counsellors, etc. Often professionals do not just help the person with their problems and bad situations, they teach them problem-solving skills (e.g. Nezu, Nezu, & D'Zurilla, 2007; Stillmaker & Kassser, 2013). There are some general methods proposed for solving problems but only some get enough descriptions of the contexts and how they fit together (de Shazer, 1988). Other therapists have always been open to making changes more

Table 5.1 Conflicts in everyday life and some intervention ideas

Life situation problem	Conflict	Intervention ideas
Too much stress in obtaining life resources (resources in a broad sense)	Blockages from resources	Work to unblock or find alternative resources, reduce need for this particular resource
	Limited opportunities	Find equal opportunities or ways to avoid blockages, find ways to use alternatives
	Lacking life skills needed	Identify skills, possibly from others, and train
	Needs extensive stories to obtain	Work with person to reduce need for stories, sharpen their stories, make stories more persuasive, less complex and likely to trap, more coherent or consistent
Too much stress in life social relationships	Social conflicts	Resolve conflicts
	Competing relationships	Remove competition and facilitate cooperation and sharing
	Pressure of image management for social relationships	Change or stop image management, or work to create doable images
	Lacking the social skills needed	Identify skills, possibly from others, and train
	Serious language confusions from audience pressures	Trace audiences for each language or thinking set, change verbal behaviour or train new verbal behaviour
	Needs extensive stories to manage competing relationships	Trace audiences for stories, work out which parts of stories are necessary or can be pruned, build new parts of stories if needed for relationships, change audiences if needed, provide new or more consistent audiences, make stories less complex and likely to trap

Conflicting ways of obtaining resources	Competing sources	Stop competition, find alternative resources, reduce need for this particular resource
	Competing opportunities	Find other opportunities that are less competitive and with less conflict, reduce need for this particular resource
	Lacking the skills needed	Identify skills, possibly from others, and train, train negotiation and conflict resolution skills
	Needs extensive stories to mitigate conflict	Work with person to reduce need for stories, sharpen stories, make stories more persuasive, less complex and likely to trap, more coherent or consistent
Conflicting audiences and social relationships	Producing strongly conflicting thoughts and thinking patterns from negotiating	Train to be ok with conflicting thoughts, train for a consistent story, defuse the conflict of stories, produce a third version of stories
	Conflicting audiences brought together somehow	Prevent audiences being together, work on new stories for both audiences, detach from stories altogether for one or both audiences
	Lacking the skills needed	Identify skills, possibly from others, and train, train relationship skills and conflict resolution skills
	Serious language confusions arising from conflicting audiences	Make stories more coherent and consistent where possible, reduce the need to tell stories, reduce the ownership of stories, trace and place stories on to the audience's previous responses not the thinker
	Needs extensive stories to mitigate conflict	Work with person to reduce need for stories, sharpen stories, make stories more persuasive, less complex and likely to trap, more coherent or consistent

(*continued*)

Table 5.1 Cont.

Life situation problem	Conflict	Intervention ideas
Strategies out of control or locked in	Bluff games gone wrong	Find out the stakes and reduce, provide more behavioural options, find options to back down and keep face, reduce need or worry over keeping face
	Bluff games using relationships (includes double binds)	Find out the stakes and why something other than the relationship was not used, find options to back down and keep face, reduce need or worry over keeping face
	Competition gone wrong	Change potential outcomes, stop competition for all parties, find alternative resources, reduce need for this particular resource
	Social traps escalating badly	Find out stakes and provide alternative sources, find out if keeping face is being used as resource and change this, reduce need for the resources involved
	Lacking the skills needed	Find out the games being used and train in skills to mitigate the game, train to recognize games and traps as they are beginning
	Multiple thoughts produced from strategies that might be conflicting or confusing	Trace the audiences for the thoughts about strategies that are worrying, provide new thoughts through 'therapist' as audience, produce third type of story if there are games with two interlocked agents
	Needs extensive stories to make strategies work	Work with person to reduce need for stories, sharpen stories, make stories more cooperative and les competitive or bullying, less complex and likely to trap, more coherent or consistent

directly in a person's life (with permission) when necessary and have them change their environments (Haley, 1973, 1985, 1991). Once again, when we start to focus less on the person and their 'mind' and more on bad and emerging bad situations, we will be able to do more before the situations become chronic and good solutions are blocked.

The following are some very general statements about professionals but that might also guide you, even though I know there are exceptions to all of these.

Social workers

Social workers have usually spent more time than other professionals with people *in their own world* and helped them more 'on the ground' to solve their life problems and bad situations. However, a lot of this now falls to 'carers' who again, spend more with the people and help them on real problems. This is not social workers' fault, but a consequence of modernity (V5.3). People's life problems have moved from interpersonal resource problems with family and friends, to problems with stranger social relationships and economic resourcing. To solve these now requires going through strangers and bureaucratic procedures—courts, police, local authorities, health systems, government agencies, mediators—basically, whoever is making and adjudicating the rules enforced by society to control our lives. For this (good) reason, social workers have a large part of their work now based around helping people with their problems by guiding them through these modern bureaucracies, because 'interpersonal problems' now mostly refers to stranger relationships (e.g. Chenoweth & McAuliffe, 2008; Dunk-West, 2013; Seabury, Seabury, & Garwin, 2011).

Nurses and mental health nurses

Nurses and mental health nurses often know the 'clients' well because, ironically, they spend more time talking with them informally than do psychiatrists and clinical psychologists, but they do not get to participate in their life contexts as much as social workers or carers, and are not usually allowed to get involved with bureaucratic 'authorities' to change the person's bad situation. (A recent conversation with a friend who is a mental health nurse has suggested that this is wrong, at least now. Nurses are often made now to work with clients in central and protected rooms with just windows looking out, so there is less 'real' contact with clients and their life situations.)

Psychiatrists and psychologists

Most psychiatrists and psychologists do not deal with solving the local conflicts of resources and social relationships because, as laid out in

Chapter 2, it is only when things become worse and the bad contexts from which the problems arise are hidden or generalized, that problems even get labelled as 'psychological' or 'mental health' issues. But if more time was spent earlier on working out how to solve these local problems of life ('pro-dromal analysis of bad situations'), we might prevent even worse bad situations developing.

Social anthropologists, community psychologists, counsellors, and life coaches

As part of their normal practice, most social anthropologists and commu-nity psychologists also spend time helping people directly with the local bad situations in their lives, trying to find solutions, as do social workers. Counsellors often do also but usually not outside their clinics. Like most psychiatrists and clinical psychologists, they are made to keep 'professional boundaries', which ironically prevents them finding more out about context. While there is a lot of criticism made of 'life coaches' and the lack of con-trol of their qualifications, you can perhaps now see that they are filling a role that other professionals no longer can. They help people on the ground to fix bad life situations early by directly changing their situations in prac-tical and tangible ways. Other professionals should think of them as filling the gaps they do not (or cannot) fill and change their own practice to help more broadly.

The point of these generalized comments is that once we recognize 'mental health' as a situational problem, (1) the types of interventions change, (2) the people with useful skills change, (3) preventing 'mental health' issues looks very different to the current conceptions, and (4) pre-vention of the worse outcomes actually looks *much more realistic* than a model in which you are, in theory at least, attempting to stop a brain from deteriorating. Furthermore, treating and changing bad life situations *dir-ectly* means that we can also draw upon the expertise of those who have tackled the 'non-mental health' issues (outlined earlier) that also arise from bad life situations (e.g. crime, drug taking, lying, exploitation, disaffected youth, rebels, violence, etc.).

What do Western therapists currently do?

The principal method for almost all psychotherapies and counselling now is *talking*, although psychiatrists also use *drug medication* (sadly, a lot of their talking is just to focus the medications). This predominant role of talking is often overlooked since it is so ubiquitous and taken for granted. It also clearly works to help people to some extent, although this is difficult to judge. What is less clear is what talking is doing to people in psychotherapy and counselling, and how it might effect change in their bad situations when it does. If we need to change the bad life situations people are experiencing, how does talking in an office with a stranger once a week help, at least sometimes?

To look closer at what psychologists actually do, I reviewed 19 psychotherapies and extracted their goals and what they actually do from their writings, some writings by others about them, and from DVDs of them practising (see Guerin, 2017 for details, including a comparison with what social workers actually do). I then removed the jargon and put them into more observable terms, since the jargon was extensive but disguised the similarities (the original paper has more about these 'translations'). Once this was done, most of the therapies became very similar in what they actually did, but each put more emphasis on one or more parts of therapy than did the others. But by far the major differences between the therapies was only in the theories and the jargon used (Guerin, 2017).

Overall, the main thrust of almost all the Western therapies was to do the following:

- Form a working relationship with a stranger.
- Solve small (local) problems in their life but only those that are amenable within an office.
- Act as a new audience to train some new behaviours that might change things outside the office.
- Elicit the person's talk and thinking around the problems and suffering they have.
- Attempt to act as a new audience to change those discourses (thoughts and talk) in ways that should be beneficial and reduce the suffering.

If we ignore the theoretical and jargon differences, therefore, the main thrust to learn from this is that being in an office with a stranger for a relatively short time can potentially change the person's bad environment in three ways:

- Talk them through some less serious bad situations to try and solve them, involving fairly direct resource and social relationship conflicts.
- Act as a new audience and try and shape them into new ways of behaving in their conflict situations, even though this training is done away from the actual situation and without the other players (so only role modelling and other methods are used).
- Try and change the way they talk and think about their conflict situations and hope that talk has an effect on their behaviour back in the original

context (reframing and similar practices), and try and stop their negative thinking or shape it into new thinking patterns, partly as distraction and partly in the hope that the new talking or thinking will control their later behaviour *in situ* (even though this is not guaranteed, V4.4).

So somewhere between all these, most psychotherapies seem to have some good effects in changing people's local bad situations, even if the beneficial effects have no relations to the theories being promulgated. A lot probably depends on how strong the *in-context* social shaping has been and whether in their bad situation they are strongly blocked from such new responses. But if the person has a somewhat functioning life and some resource–social relationship pathways then this might be all that is required. So, using thought-stopping and distraction methods from CBT and other methods might be all that is required for them to put up with minor bad situations if that is all they want, although the same might be gained from both religious methods and life distractions such as entertainment, etc. Wait for their situations to change naturally.

The next step from the present analysis is to leave the office and go into the person's world to try and make changes by more directly involving the other people and resource bases in the person's life. Some of this is actually done in family therapies, Indigenous therapies, and feminist therapies (more on these last two later).

What happens when you cannot talk about the problems?

We frequently see in the media that a research study has just shown that some 'activity X' leads to improved mental health: "Media release: tree hugging leads to improvements in depression". I am not disparaging this, apart from any such research that uses methods that are not really robust. Some, however, have better research programmes, such as music and art therapies, and some are starting to get more, such as walking as therapy, meditation, and mindfulness. For other we still have no research but just stories of positive outcomes, such as going to concerts, taking part in performances, surfing, tree hugging, heavy metal music therapy (Quinn, 2019), travel, nature walks, learning to be a clown, skydiving, and a range of many others.

My problem is not so much the lack of evidence, but that currently most of these do no *analysis* of what might be affecting a person's lifeworld when they do these activities, especially how these activities might improve their bad situations. They still assume that (1) the change is made 'within' the person and (2) the activity is what led to this change. In fact, every one of these I have seen involves a huge number of changes to the person's life contexts, and in many cases I doubt that the named activity itself is what is bringing about these changes. The following are typical changes and any one of these might lead to 'mental health improvement' and not the activity by itself (yes, even tree hugging!):

* Getting out of the house.
* Doing a new activity.
* Some change has already led the person to carry this out *at all*, and *how that was done* might be the strongest force in itself (Guerin, 2005).
* Removing the person from their normal contexts in which their common bad situations take place.
* Contact with new people.
* New life possibilities coming from meeting new people (resource–social relationship pathways).
* Provision of new stories and other discourses for their normal audiences about this new activity.
* Useful new discourses gained from listening to those involved in the new activity (could be advice, alternative possibilities, stories about others in similar bad situations).
* More engagement in life in a general sense.

Therapy by going for a regular walk, for example, usually includes most of the above (cf. Janet, 1919/1925). Mindfulness includes many of these (including the third point above; that if someone like a therapist can get the depressed person to actually do mindfulness training, then that in itself is a behavioural activation technique, and *this* could be more of what leads to a positive effect than the actual mindfulness procedures themselves). Hugging trees must provide many alternative self-identity discourses to tell people back in the original bad life context, and this will change how those people then interact with the tree hugger in the future and that in turn will change their social relationships.

Notice that many of these involve changing our social relationships or making new ones. I have frequently heard from people with first-hand experience that making 'social connections' was vitally important in helping them through their bad situations. It must be kept in mind that social relationships need to be seen as part of resource–social relationship pathways, and that is what is gained by 'social connectedness'. Not just someone to talk to, but someone to connect to resources and opportunities, even in small ways.

So, I am not arguing that these activities do *not* have effects, just that the named activity itself (tree hugging, mindfulness) is not what necessarily leads to any changes. The problem is that with so many ways it might work, being successful for one person or for one bad situation does not mean it will work for others. Only observations in context will tell us.

There is one other facet to all these 'alternative' approaches to therapy that might also be beneficial. We have seen (V4.6, V4.7) that there are *gaps between using language and the actual world itself*. There are experiences we have and things we do that *cannot* be put into words, so talking therapies fail at this point. The therapy context calls for *some* sort of response, and the usual responses that occur when these situations arise are the behaviours we call 'emotional' (V4.6). And because 'mental health' behaviours are defined by their contexts being hidden, this will occur frequently.

So, therapy requires ways of dealing with such contexts, although the usual procedure is to (1) let the person experience the emotional responses and try to get them to talk about it later (bordering on contradiction), and (2) present them with the therapist's *theories* about what is happening when they cannot respond in words (Guerin, 2019b). But humans have other ways to respond that might lead to changes in their bad situations, including music, poetry, painting, drawing, and dancing, and some of the 'alternative' therapies given earlier might also function well in such non-word contexts. Some like music therapy already have good evidence that starts to look at the question of how playing, listening to, or composing music can change a person's bad situations in some way that is therapeutic (Ansdell, 2014; DeNora, 2015; Guerin, 2019a, 2020; Quinn, 2019; Rowe, 2018; Rowe & Guerin, 2018).

References

Ansdell, G. (2014). *How music helps in music therapy and everyday life*. London: Routledge.

Chenoweth, L., & McAuliffe, D. (2012). *The road to social work & human service practice*. Melbourne: Cenage Learning.

de Shazer, S. (1988). *Clues: Investigating solutions in brief therapy*. New York, NY: W. W. Norton.

DeNora, T. (2015). *Music asylums: Wellbeing through music in everyday life*. London: Routledge.

Dunk-West, P. (2013). *How to be a social worker: A critical guide for students*. New York, NY: Palgrave Macmillan.

Gluckman, M. (1965). *Politics, law and ritual in tribal society*. Oxford: Basil Blackwell.

Gluckman, M. (Ed.) (1972). *The allocation of responsibility*. Manchester: Manchester University Press.

Guerin, B. (2005). *Handbook of interventions for changing people and communities*. Reno, NV: Context Press.

Guerin, B. (2017). Deconstructing psychological therapies as activities in context: What are the goals and what do therapists actually do? *Revista Perspectivas em Análise do Comportamento, 8*, 97–119.

Guerin, B. (2019a). Contextualizing music to enhance music therapy. *Revista Perspectivas em Anályse Comportamento*, *10*, 222–242.

Guerin, B. (2019b). What do therapists and clients talk about when they cannot explain behaviours? How Carl Jung avoided analysing a client's environments by inventing theories. *Revista Perspectivas em Anályse Comportamento*, *10*, 76–97.

Guerin, B. (2020). What does poetry do to readers and listeners, and how does it do this? Language use as social activity and its clinical relevance. *Revista Brasileira de Análise do Comportamento*, *15*.

Haley, J. (1973). *Uncommon therapy: The psychiatric techniques of Milton H. Erickson, M.D.* London: Norton.

Haley, J. (Ed.) (1985). *Conversations with Milton H. Erickson, M.D. Volume 1: Changing individuals.* New York, NY: Triangle Press.

Haley, J. (1991). *Problem-solving therapy.* New York, NY: Jossey-Bass.

Janet, P. (1919/1925). *Psychological healing: A historical and clinical study.* London: George Allen & Unwin.

Johnstone, L., Boyle, M., Cromby, J., Dillon, J., Harper, D., Kinderman, P., … Read, J. (2018). *The Power Threat Meaning Framework: Towards the identification of patterns in emotional distress, unusual experiences and troubled or troubling behaviour, as an alternative to functional psychiatric diagnosis.* Leicester: British Psychological Society.

Mills, C. W. (1959). *The sociological imagination.* Oxford: Oxford University Press.

Nezu, A. M., Nezu, C. M., & D'Zurilla, T. J. (2007). *Solving life's problems: A 5-step guide to enhanced wellbeing.* New York, NY: Springer.

Quinn, K. (2019). Heavy metal music and managing mental health: Heavy metal therapy. *Metal Music Studies*, *5*, 419–424.

Roberts, S. (1979). *Order and dispute: An introduction to legal anthropology.* Harmondsworth, UK: Penguin.

Rowe, P. (2018). *Heavy metal youth identities: Researching the musical empowerment of youth transitions and psychosocial wellbeing.* London: Emerald Publishing.

Rowe, P., & Guerin, B. (2018). Contextualizing the mental health of metal youth: A community for social protection, identity and musical empowerment. *Journal of Community Psychology*, *46*, 1–13.

Schwartz, A., & Goldiamond, I. (1975). *Social casework: A behavioral approach.* New York, NY: Columbia University Press.

Seabury, B. A., Seabury, B. H., & Garwin, C. D. (2011). *Foundations of interpersonal practice in social work: Promoting competence in generalist practice.* New York, NY: Sage

Stillmaker, J., & Kasser, T. (2013). Instruction in problem-solving skills increases the hedonic balance of highly neurotic individuals. *Cognitive Therapy and Research*, *37*, 380–382.

Watson, J. (2019). *Drop the disorder: Challenging the culture of psychiatric diagnosis.* London: PCCS Books.

6   How can we change language use and thinking in 'mental health'?

Partly because of the ubiquity of language and thinking (V4) in our modern lives—using language is the main way we make things happen in life—and partly because therapy itself has become overwhelmingly about talking (cf. Janet, 1919/1925), we need to look closely at how language and thinking figure in bad situations and their outcomes. Psychology focuses upon CBT, but 'cognitive', as I have stressed (V4.8), is really about language use, and the social relationships and social exchanges that allow language to function at all.

There are four main ways in which language use enters into 'mental health' once we understand that language (both talking and thinking) arise externally in our social and discursive worlds. First, language uses arise from difficult-to-see social contexts, so people often behave in non-useful ways when dealing with their problems through language. Second, therapists primarily use language to intervene. Third, talking in bad situations often gets punished because of the first point, and so these discourses become thought rather than said out loud (V4.4). Finally, we primarily solve problems and change our worlds through other people via talking. This means that when things go bad our first solution attempts will be discursive—getting other people to do something different by telling or asking them—and these will also get punished frequently unless the situations get solved.

So, the point is that both talking and thinking issues (formerly known as 'disorders') are really issues with trying to change people (family, friends, strangers, bureaucrats) in order to change your bad situations. They are not about hidden away processes in your mind, mental processes, or 'cognitive processing', they are about social relationships. When you encounter talking and thinking problems, they are problems with someone trying to shift their world via their social relationships (see the 'lettuce' example in Box 6.1).

The history of therapies, therefore (see Chapter 1), is replete with problems of thinking and 'thought disorders', but I argue that *thinking problems really disguise problems arising from trying to change other people to change bad life situations but the relationships are messed up.* This is now especially difficult when trying to change what strangers do (V2, V5.3), so living in modernity where stranger relationships increasingly predominate, 'thinking' problems are more and more common. And indeed, from Janet and Freud onwards, a strong focus has been on thoughts and their role in 'mental illness' even though the real basis for this are the new dilemmas of stranger social relationships rather than any problems with the brain per se.

Talking and thought 'disorders' are therefore really about social relationships falling apart (see Chapter 5), and this is increasingly frequent with the plethora of stranger relationships we require in modernity to get all the resources we need. *When someone is not doing well with social relationships*, especially with strangers or trying to find a balance between the family and strangers in their lives, then their discourses will fall apart. The effects of this can be seen in the following:

- Language and thinking becoming divorced from getting resources or doing productive actions ('dissociation').
- Exaggerated talking and thinking (both in intensity from silence to shouting, and in content and how it affects listeners).
- 'Existential' issues that break any coherent and consistent self-stories (V5.5).
- The poor use of beliefs that could hold their world together, including both lack of beliefs and rigid beliefs (V5.4).
- Problems with 'me' thoughts and thinking becoming dissociated.

The first historical approach in modern therapy was to try and get the person to say their hidden (punished) thoughts out loud, with many believing that this alone would change things or produce a 'cure' (Freud, counselling, etc.). But 'catharsis' through talking, when it seems to work, is still about changing bad external social situations not 'internal' situations (Guerin, 2001, V5.1). The second approach in modernity has been to either distract the person from bad thoughts, or to try and shape ('reframe') new thoughts to replace those bad ones (CBT, hypnosis, narrative therapies, etc.). The limits to the success of these has often been said to be the strength of the thoughts or beliefs, but I contend that it is the strength with which the bad situations of social relationships and discursive communities have shaped those thoughts in the first place—how much you 'need' those thoughts to keep your social relationships and hence your resources (V5.4, V5.5).

But there are centuries of other methods for dealing with talking and thinking, including non-word methods involving the performance of arts to change bad situations, and the use of practices such as prayer, meditation, and chanting. As we saw in the last chapter (with tree hugging), these might be effective through many pathways, and most include the CBT goals of distraction or reframing. At the same time, many also involve a lot of social support and direct action in solving crises, and once again just getting the person to do these activities might alone be beneficial, especially when thinking problems are really social relationship problems in disguise (V4.4).

Next, I will briefly go through a few general points about modern Western methods, and then a little of what we know about other practices such as prayer, meditation, and chanting (see also Guerin, 2017).

Some points about thoughts in modern Western therapy

From all the above there are important things to note about therapies, which, like our social relationships, are primarily about talking to have effects in the client's world.

1. First, it is important to focus on the following:
   - What we say.
   - What we can report as our thoughts.
   - What we report as our thoughts with some questioning and contextualizing.

   Around any problematic issue in life there can be thoughts that we can *easily report* (conscious) and some that are *difficult to report* but once stated out loud we can agree that they were thoughts we 'had' all along (unconscious). The differences between these are not in the thoughts themselves but in their *social conditions* (whether they have been punished out loud or not, etc., see V4.4).

   The important point is that all these are good clues in therapy for understanding people's conflicts and issues in life around social relationships, which then can be addressed in many ways (changing the client's verbal responses is only one of the ways therapists can work).

2. One role of a therapist, therefore, is to *create those social contexts in which reporting thoughts of all kinds is easier*, especially those thoughts that are punished in many social situations if said out loud. There are many ways of doing this—from psychoanalysis, non-directive therapies, Gestalt therapy, dialectical behaviour therapy (DBT), acceptance and commitment therapy (ACT), etc., as well as prayer and some forms of meditation.

3. There are interesting cases in which a thought will occur to someone or even be said out loud, but *in any or all situations* in their life rather than

just in the relevant contexts (obsessions, dysfunctional cognitions). We must look to observe the *social contexts* that make this generalization happen, not the nature or content of those thoughts (which could actually be irrelevant)

4. In many therapies, questioning soon finishes with only the reporting of any out loud talk ("So when she said that, I replied to her that ..."). Better therapies get into the *unsaid verbal responses* in difficult or conflict situations, and *contextualize the social relationship issues from which the talking and thinking problems arise*:

    *   What were you thinking at that point?
    *   How were you feeling about that?
    *   What were you thinking about that at the time?
    *   What else were you thinking about at the time?
    *   What would you have liked to have said at that point?

5. The following extract is Freud talking to a client, and tracing through questioning some of the context around her 'belief' that she loves her employer:

> She answered in her usual laconic fashion: "Yes, I think that's true"—"But if you knew you loved your employer why didn't you tell me!"—"I didn't know—or rather I didn't want to know. I wanted to drive it out of my head and not think of it again; and I believe latterly I have succeeded." "Why was it that you were unwilling to admit this inclination? Were you ashamed of loving a man?"—"Oh no, I'm not unreasonably prudish. We're not responsible for our feelings, anyhow. It was distressing to me only because he is my employer and I am in his service and live in his house. I don't feel the same complete independence towards him that I could towards anyone else. And then I am only a poor girl and he is such a rich man of good family. People would laugh at me if they had any idea of it."
>
> (Breuer & Freud, 1895/1974, pp. 181–182)

Freud managed to get at the unsaid thoughts that she earlier could not report and dredge up some *social, economic, and cultural context* at the same time, relevant to her life problems (Pathway 2). However, he later added a lot of theoretical terms to 'help explain' these natural events (Pathway 1).

6. Some therapies spend more time questioning clients for the *unsaid verbal responses* that have been shaped in their clients' lives, but that are only rarely spoken out loud or not at all by those clients. For example:

Box 6.1 Discourse analysis of a 'psychotic' example of discourse (SALADA)

Here is an example of 'word salad', a term once used to describe some language uses lumped into the 'schizophrenia' diagnosis. Read it first and then try analysing yourself. I will then discuss common analyses and a discourse analysis procedure (although this is historical so we cannot find out more now about this person). I will try to illustrate that 'word salad' is not 'disorganized thought and speech': like any discourse it is all about *doing* things to people with language use.

> Interviewer: Have you been nervous or tense lately?
> John: No, I got a head of lettuce.
> Interviewer: You got a head of lettuce? I don't understand.
> John: Well, it's just a head of lettuce.
> Interviewer: Tell me about the lettuce. What do you mean?
> John: Well ... Lettuce is a transformation of a dead cougar that suffered a relapse on the lion's toe. And he swallowed the lion and something happened. The ... see, the... Gloria and Tommy, they're two heads and they're not whales. But they escaped with herds of vomit, and things like that.
>
> (Neale & Oltmanns, 1980)

Typical analyses

Most people hearing this try *interpreting* what the person (speaking the word salad) *really meant*: what was the person trying to *express*? What was the person trying to *communicate*? What was the person trying to *refer to* or *represent*? The interviewer asks about 'meaning', for example.

Discourse analysis (SALADA)

First, we must look at the social analysis (SA). The person being interviewed, from the little that we know:

- was trapped in an 'asylum';
- obviously had many life conflicts and bad situations they had not yet solved;
- had been interned some time so obviously they were not really being helped;
- was constantly being asked questions by clinicians;
- was expected to say all the normal boring and superficial things of good middle-class conversation;

- had to tell the interviewer that everything was okay when it was not;
- was controlled by the clinician as to when they would be released.

Second, what were some of the language aspects (linguistic analysis, LA) and the possible social strategies that were going on *in context* (discourse analysis, DA)?

- This particular conversation was *started* by the psychologist/ psychiatrist.
- The psychologist/psychiatrist asked if they were nervous or tense, probably for the hundredth time.
- Asking if they are nervous or tense is a ridiculous question because obviously the person is not okay. It is also a ridiculous question to ask someone locked up and having their life controlled by an institution.
- Unlike ourselves in this conversational situation (of people asking stupid questions), the client could not just exit the situation, avoid that relationship ever again, or laugh it off with a joke like we might; these options are blocked.
- If the client had just been rude or abrasive, this would have caused further problems for them, including extra diagnoses from acting 'aggressive' or 'oppositional'.
- So what might this 'word salad' have actually *been doing* to the psychologist?
- What might it *do* within the social context of this interview and relationship, how did it function?
- From a sociolinguistic perspective, the patient was breaking all of Grice's 'maxims' of polite conversation and wrecking all the adjacency pairs, and this is usually done to have the effect of *breaking off* or *diminishing the social relationship*.
- They also were presenting abstract and obfuscating answers to deflect inquiries, challenges, normal conversation, and relationship building.
- The client did this *perfectly* by talking word salad, which makes sense when you put it in this sort of context.

That is, you need to think about what this language is *doing* in the situation, to try and change the client's bad situation of being locked up and controlled, in addition to whatever original bad things occurred. If you do this, then it was perfectly formed to stop, escape, or diminish the social relationship and conversation with the listener. In this functional sense, it was not 'disorganized' at all!

Other interventions for 'mental health' issues involving talking and thinking

When we think of interventions to help with the behaviours we currently call 'mental health' issues, most people think of psychotherapies and psychiatry. However, there have been numerous other ways in which people have dealt with these issues over centuries. If 'mental illnesses' were really about brain diseases then many of these other interventions could be called 'superstitious', and indeed they have been called that (V5.1). But if we treat our behaviours in a new way, as suggested in Chapter 2, then these practices make a lot of sense whether or not you believe in the underlying theology or scriptures. We will look at just a few of these in this chapter.

For this chapter we need to go back to Chapter 2 and the varieties of thinking. We saw there that most of what we call 'thinking' is simply talking in a mostly normal way, responding to all the conversations and discourses around us during our lives, and influencing people. However, for a number of reasons outlined earlier (V4, Table 4.1), we do not speak some of these discourses out loud and so they are called thinking rather than talking. The differences between the two are not differences in kind, but differences arising from (1) the specific contexts for *not* saying them out loud in the first place, and (2) the lack of consequences because they will not be heard and responded to by real people.

The second point is that there are gaps in the world between what we can say (to affect people) and what really happens in what we do and experience (V4.7). Saying "I saw a dog" or "I see a triangle" (V4.1) are great for affecting people in real social life, but they are not good descriptions of what has taken place nor of your actual experience. There are serious gaps.

The point of this here is that in bad situations especially there are many things we do or experience that *cannot* be said adequately in words, and especially not using our normal social discourses that are only there to affect someone to do something. This means that both to describe experiences and also to affect people to help change situations, words do not always suffice. We can substitute more physical actions in such cases (to try and change our worlds via people), or we can try and affect people with *activities that not involve words directly* (music, dance, arts, hand movements, etc.).

So, in summary, I will look at a few methods outside typical Western psychotherapies, with which we can distract or block thoughts, reframe thoughts, get thoughts said out loud that might have been punished (V4.4, Box 4.1), or change our audiences without even using words (Hadot, 1995; Siedentop, 2014).

Prayers and praying

When you sit in silence, in a marae, cathedral, mosque, or any room alone, you might hear voices or 'thinking'. They are all from the discourses from all around your lifeworlds, but they are unique to you since no one else will have the same. Each of them is from a part of your life (even slogans from TV adverts) and if you can 'catch' them, *they are usually the ones of importance*—whether a good or a bad influence and direction. It is your discernment whether to use them and talk about new pathways with these voices.

See the problem? In everyday life we are not hearing all these but each thought or voice is from a part of your life situation and is telling us many things we do not hear. We tend to just hear the one critical and rational voice arguing against whatever is being said, as if in verbal competition. The others are not irrational, they are just from other audiences, other sources, other discourses than our critical voice 'listens to' normally (V5.1). And whether or not you believe the stories of the origin of these voices and sounds, all of them are a very useful and valuable resource to use in your life. And this is usually wasted for most people nowadays, until it is too late.

These voices or thoughts are literally discussing your life from different perspectives, since they arose from your different audiences and sources. If you fight with someone and leave, you will have a flurry of 'conversations' going on. If you are daydreaming you will hear things people said, things you said, things said on television, and things you would like to have said but did not. These get wasted unless 'heard', and they can be valuable. Some you do not want to 'hear', like someone telling you that you should do X instead of doing Y, but this can be valuable to you to *consider* even if you still do Y. And especially when you are in a bad situation, it can be valuable to consider all these things 'floating in your thoughts'.

So many of the methods for handling bad situations and thinking include (1) distractions, (2) reframing, (3) 'listening' to all the 'hidden' discourses and finding ways to respond if they help the situation, and (4) placing the thoughts into the contexts of the bad situation to see how they might be functioning (if said out loud). Freud did this with free association and his other methods, and prayers and chanting can do likewise, as can using dreams (Graham, 1995; Marett, 2005; Rasmussen, 2015; Tedlock, 1987).

The social contexts for praying, chanting, and recitation

There are many effects of praying and many ways of doing praying (e.g. Ulanov & Ulanov, 1982; Zaleski & Zaleski, 2005). I will talk about just a few here but there is so much more to be explored. Most also include an increase in social and community contact, and as we saw in Chapter 5, this on its own can assist in getting out of bad situations (e.g. my tree-hugging example).

One of the first big distinctions in praying is between the use of praying to request or plea for help in some matters or praying just to hear the many discourses or voices floating around in your life. The former has always occurred, pleading to greater powers (the environmental elements as well) for health, wealth, or something else. This can have many social effects even if unsuccessful. Praying in general can help articulate thoughts but still without saying them out loud. If saying something was punished so it is not said out loud, 'praying' is like saying the words out loud to someone or something. This is no different to Freud's methods really, of getting people to speak out loud *to him* their 'hidden' (punished) discourses. This can be helpful in many ways socially without getting punished. Because these unsaid thoughts are usually about the most difficult parts of our life discourses, this gives an opportunity to produce innovative ways to respond verbally to old conflict situations.

Praying to hear the unsaid discourses in your life (or discourses from God if you prefer) is a very different practice and some religions and groups do not allow this. Catholicism, for example, has not allowed people to talk directly with God and instead people must listen to a priest's sermon or chant and incant words from scriptures and hymns. Many who said they heard God talk directly to them were persecuted. Jeanne d'Arc in the fifteenth century was put to death for claiming to hear some of the saints speak directly to her. However, other Christian churches and other religions allow, or even encourage, a person to hear God's voice directly.

Chanting and recitation, on the other hand, *provide* the words rather than give the silence to hear all the floating unsaid discourses about our life situations. These practices can help both by *distraction* (much the same as some CBT), and by *providing new discourses* that might be of benefit (as a therapist tries to do in reframing and other methods).

On the other hand, the *difficulties* with prayer are: what to do with all the discourses one hears when praying? Do you ignore some, ignore all, choose some for your focus, or what? The *difficulty* with chanting and recitation comes from either the distraction not working or from the verses chosen not having any benefit. Most of these practices, therefore, are somewhat hit and miss and not every session of prayer leads to a life change—but the same can be said about all the psychotherapies.

When we look at these practices we must remember that there are already social and other contexts present for the events to take place (again, just like psychotherapies). If people are helped and change from the events this does not mean that the events that took place were the cause or instigation of change: the contexts that brought the events about could have done that (Guerin, 2005). For example, in a Somali community I was working alongside, when someone was not themselves (including having what we call 'mental health issues'), some of the community and the imam would organize Koran readings. This would bring together the troubled person to have readings from specific parts of the Koran appropriate to that issue. The point here is to remember that *making* these readings happen and the community involvement specifically for a person in trouble, might have been, on their own, enough to bring about some change in behaviour (Guerin, 2005).

Finally, these analyses do not depend upon the truth of the words used to talk about praying. I am analysing from just one perspective—social contextual analysis—but analyses in terms of theology are equally welcome. One of my goals is to show atheists and agnostics that the events are not shams and they can be the locus of some important behavioural changes. This is regardless of whether you think about the events of praying and chanting in religious or spiritual terms, and indeed I believe the theories and stories given by current therapies and psychiatry are similar. I will leave that to the reader. For example, when sitting in silence at a Quaker meeting, the discourses, voices, and fragments of silent talking are important for the person, whether or not you believe these voices are (1) previous discourses left unsaid that are important in your life (V4.4); or (2) God talking directly to you, 'nudging' you into certain ways of deciding and acting (see examples in Box 6.2).

Music

We saw earlier that when there are problematic issues to which we must respond but we have no learned responses, then music is one form of behaviour that is often done in lieu of speaking (Guerin, 2019). Music can give us some responses rather than none, it can distract us from the problems, and it can provide us with social events to talk about in negotiating our identities and resources through social relationships.

> If I could express the same thing with words as with music, I would, of course, use a verbal expression. Music is something autonomous and much richer. Music begins where the possibilities of language end. That is why I write music.
>
> (Sibelius, 1919)

Box 6.2 Quaker discernment

There is a really interesting Quaker tradition of listening to our 'voices' and working *with* those voices. They call it 'discernment'. For Quakers, in such a process one must first hear all the voices from sources that we cannot see and then discern which are from God and which are from your own 'ego' (V4.4). Discernment leads to better decision-making and Quakers have procedures for doing this in groups, because they dislike or mistrust procedures of basic consensus.

> We believe that God speaks with us all the time, whispering in our ears, nudging our emotions, stirring our senses, and drawing us to the preferred path. Even now, as you read these words, God may be stirring within you, calling, opening, and speaking to you. God desires to be your partner, to journey through life with you.
>
> Both God and humans seek the reality of this dialogue and companionship. Spiritual discernment is the process of learning the language and the process of this relationship.
>
> (Fendall et al., 2007, p. 23)

For those who do not believe in a God this is still very important for our lives, and we can think about it in the terms I am presenting in this book instead. I experienced this unexpectedly powerful way of tracking your thoughts and the external contexts from which they arise came when I visited a Quaker meeting in Pennsylvania. The main 'service' consists of sitting in silence with anywhere from 50 to 100 other people while 'listening to your thoughts'. Part of the Quaker's process is to 'discern' whether the voices you hear come from God, your own 'ego', or from other people.

For me, a strong part of the experience *was having the other people in the room* with you all sitting in silence. This was very, very different to sitting in a room all by yourself meditating or contemplating your navel. Having the other people in the room highlighted social relationships and greatly enhanced the voices (thoughts, unsaid language responses). The presence of people also made it easier to differentiate your usual voice (your habitual language responses that you use in most of your social relationships) from the other voices that normally you do not notice.

Or as Ansdell put it:

> We suggest that music doesn't have some magical power in itself, but rather that what music can uniquely do shows up *between* people, *within* situations, and *about* specific local needs and possibilities. Music comes to life and quickens others only within and amongst a musical ecology.
>
> (Ansdell, 2014, p. xvi)

Music is a social event and can change other people and hence your own bad situations, without any words (of course much music combines both, "The answer, my friend is ..."). Like all the above, it can entertain and distract from bad thoughts and situations, it can change situations, it can change other people to change your bad situation, and it can provide new discourses through lyrics. Usually it gives little opportunity to hear the 'hidden' discourses, however.

So like painting, poetry, and dance, playing, listening to, or composing music provides a context for many possible changes in events to occur. But it is especially useful when words and changing other people through words is just not working (Guerin, 2019, 2020; Quinn, 2019; Rowe & Guerin, 2018).

Some examples and quotes

The following are a few quotes to consider. See whether you can think of what these are doing in terms of this book, and thinking, talking, and other discourses encountered in life that are not said out loud for various reasons:

> Some methods focus on the distractions themselves. The worshipper may invite the worries, excitements, and desires to present themselves, then gently dismiss each one, acknowledging its role in the worshipper's life and agreeing to return to them after the time of worship. Then, if these thoughts return during meeting for worship, they are recognized in advance before they have completely absorbed the worshipper's attention.
>
> (Birkel, 2004, p. 41)

> Discernment is sorting, careful listening, and recognizing. Discernment offers a tool to distinguish between an interior leading from God and an impulse whose origin is less worthy, such as a desire to feel important or look clever.
>
> (Birkel, 2004, p. 55)

No matter how much a thought may persecute you, all you have to do is let it go by. By fighting it, you stir up other thoughts ... You cannot do this prayer by willpower. The more effort you put into it, the less well it goes. When you catch yourself trying hard, relax and let go ... Of course, when thoughts are flying at you like baseballs, you look around for some means to protect yourself. But swatting them out of the park is not the way to do it. You should honestly say, "Well, I am being pummelled with these thoughts", and put up with them, remembering that if you just wait, they will all pass by.

(Keating, 1992, p. 58)

It is important to remember that human language has limitations. When we speak of "hearing God" or of "God speaking" with us, we use these words to imply physical hearing. Most often, however, God communicates with us without words that we hear with our physical ears.

(Fendall, Wood, & Bishop, 2007, p. 24)

If God is constantly stirring within us, reaching out every day to communicate and journey with us, then why do we rarely hear this communication? ... This is not necessarily a call to be less busy, but rather, less distracted. You can spend the day sitting on your couch and still not settle into the presence of God. Conversely, you can go about the demands of your day while still cultivating your attentiveness to the presence of God.

(Fendall et al., 2007, pp. 26–27)

References

Ansdell, G. (2014). *How music helps in music therapy and everyday life.* London: Routledge.

Birkel, M. L. (2004). *Silence and witness: The Quaker tradition.* New York, NY: Orbis Books.

Breuer, J., & Freud, S. (1895/1974). *Studies on hysteria* (Penguin Freud Library Volume 3). London: Penguin.

Fendall, L., Wood, J., & Bishop, B. (2007). *Practicing discernment together: Finding God's way forward in decision making.* Newberg, OR: Barclay Press

Freud, S. (1925/1984). 'Negation'. In S. Freud, *On metapsychology* (pp. 437–442) (Penguin Freud Library Volume 11). London: Penguin.

Graham, L. R. (1995). *Performing dreams: Discourses of immortality among the Xavante of Central Brazil.* Austin: University of Texas Press.

Guerin, B. (2001). Replacing catharsis and uncertainty reduction theories with descriptions of the historical and social context. *Review of General Psychology, 5,* 44–61.

Guerin, B. (2005). *Handbook of interventions for changing people and communities*. Reno, NV Context Press.

Guerin, B. (2017). *How to rethink mental illness: The human contexts behind the labels*. London: Routledge.

Guerin, B. (2019). Contextualizing music to enhance music therapy. *Revista Perspectivas em Anályse Comportamento, 10*, 222–242.

Guerin, B. (2020). What does poetry do to readers and listeners, and how does it do this? Language use as social activity and its clinical relevance. *Revista Brasileira de Análise do Comportamento, 15*.

Hadot, P. (1995). *Philosophy as a way of life: Spiritual exercises from Socrates to Foucault*. London: Blackwell.

Janet, P. (1919/1925). *Psychological healing: A historical and clinical study*. London: George Allen & Unwin.

Keating, T. (1992). *Open mind, open heart: The contemplative dimension of the gospel*. Shaftesbury, UK: Element.

Marett, A. (2005). *Songs, dreamings, and ghosts: The Wangga of North Australia*. Middletown, CO: Wesleyan University Press.

Neale, J. M., & Oltmanns, T. F. (1980). *Schizophrenia*. New York, NY: J. Wiley.

Quinn, K. (2019). Heavy metal music and managing mental health: Heavy metal therapy. *Metal Music Studies, 5*, 419–424.

Rasmussen, S. (2015). An ambiguous spirit dream and Tuareg–Kunta relationships in rural Northern Mali. *Anthropological Quarterly, 88*, 635–664.

Rowe, P., & Guerin, B. (2018). Contextualizing the mental health of metal youth: A community for social protection, identity and musical empowerment. *Journal of Community Psychology, 46*, 1–13.

Sibelius, J. (1919, 10 June). Interview with Berlingske Tidende. Retrieved from www.sibelius.fi/suomi/index.html.

Siedentop, L. (2014). *Inventing the individual: The origins of Western liberalism*. London: Penguin Books.

Tedlock, B. (Ed.) (1987). *Dreaming: Anthropological and psychological interpretations*. Santa Fe, NM: School of American Research Press.

Ulanov, A., & Ulanov, B. (1982). *Primary speech: A psychology of prayer*. Louisville, KT: Westminster John Knox Press.

Zaleski, P., & Zaleski, C. (2005). *Prayer: A history*. New York, NY: Houghton Mifflin.

7 How can we change behaviours shaped by the bad situations produced by societal structures of modernity?

One of the points of the earlier chapters was that the bad situations we encounter in life shape us into many behaviours that can eventually hurt us. Most of those bad situations, however, are not purely local but partly involve the structures of society, not only by restricting or blocking what we can do to escape or avoid such bad situations, but also by *causing the bad situations in the first place*. This applies to all human responses when put into bad situations, not just those labelled as 'mental health' issues.

If governments and authorities are serious about reducing the incidence of 'mental health' problems in society, as they profess to be in their election promises, they must now realize that the societal systems they run and promote are both causing many of the problems and also blocking solutions for people. *Many interventions for 'mental health' therefore require us to move from individual treatments to social and societal actions.*

Naomi Klein (2019, p. 31) wrote about climate change: "Climate change is a collective problem, and it demands collective action". To now paraphrase and add to this: *'Mental health' is a collective problem, and it demands collective action, even for individuals.*

Currently, Western governments treat 'mental health' following a capitalist/neoliberal agenda: that problems for citizens are individual problems and the process *must* be to: (1) identify the individual's problem through standardized assessment, (2) get a standardized (and marketable) product to change it, and (3) implement this solution (preferably one size fits all). Such agendas and processes *exclude* the proper and full treatment of both people as social beings and the government as made up of social beings not a rationality machine (V5.1).

So, the systems of society arise in 'mental health' issues as both *causing* the bad situations and *preventing* people from doing the very things they need to escape or avoid their bad situations, and therefore seriously go about reducing the incidence of 'mental health' problems in society.

Bad life problems with hidden bad situations but not considered 'mental health' issues

One of the changes in thinking suggested in this book is to stop separating 'mental health' problems from other 'problem' behaviours that have been shaped in the very same bad situations. As I have argued, they are all shaped in often hidden bad situations when most 'normal' and even alternative resource–social relationship pathways are blocked, and so to survive, extreme behaviours are shaped and these then become trapped into chronic strategies.

Examples arising in these ways not usually categorized as 'mental health' issues include domestic violence, lying and deception, 'dropping out' of mainstream practices, exploitation, bullying, crime and drug-taking. There has always been discussion over cases that could fall into either category, but I am suggesting that we should get rid of the categorization altogether and focus on *how humans respond to bad life situations*. It is also likely that successful treatments for one will help in a modified form for the others.

There are many other possible responses in bad situations that are neither violent or criminal, nor do they fall under the loose category of 'mental health'. In the last chapter (and V4.6) we saw that when bad situations are hidden or societal, then it is often difficult or impossible to talk about what is going on anyway (in order to change something). Hence, we see a number of *non-language-use responses* as well, including physical activities, music, poetry, dance, art, walking, meditation, yoga, nature experiences, mindfulness, reading, pet therapy, and travel. We also can see a number of people changing their environments by 'dropping out' or finding alternative communities that do not sit within the mainstream. Some of the above, but not all, can arise from within bad situations in an attempt to change something (Daniels, 1981; Glasper, 2006; Kaemmer, 1989; Odell, 2019; Purcell, 2003; Rowe, 2018; Rowe & Guerin, 2018; Scott-Heron, 2000; Taylor, 2017; Truong, 2018; Varas-Díaz & Scott, 2016). And sadly, another solution for many people is simply to 'put up with it'.

Bad life problems with hidden bad situations that are not considered to be 'mental health' issues

I want to add a category here, not because I believe in the categories but because they can be useful to make people more sensitive to diversities. As discussed elsewhere (V4.7), categories can never 'capture' the world so that is not their use for me. I believe their use is to get people to see *new* things they have not seen before (sensitize readers), and to then go beyond this to observe examples not covered by the category system (Deleuzian). Unlike the DSM, I do not want readers to focus on fitting life to *any* categories (V4.7), but to focus on real-life observations and experiences. And if my categories help in doing that, good. If not, ignore them.

As already mentioned (see Chapter 3), some people in bad situations 'put up with it', usually because at least some other parts of their life are okay or because they are punished more if they do not. They are therefore likely over time to develop forms of behaviours that are shaped by this life situation, those called 'mental health' issues, and others.

Many of these situations are also hidden, meaning that people often do not know why they are unhappy or anxious, they cannot observe and describe their contexts, so they are shaped to 'put up with it' and have mild forms of the behaviours outlined above (e.g. sad and depressed but not matching a 'clinical criterion'). Many of these hidden bad situations are created by the society they are living in, and most societies have ideologies, marketing, and discourses that promote that this is the only or the best way to live and that they should be followed so as to prevent things getting worse (my 'prodromal situation analysis'; see Chapter 5).

Most are shaped to reduce the suffering through the usual ways: to block or distract the suffering (entertainment); change their life discourses to make the suffering seem less to people around them; to keep the necessary social relationships going (reframing, and alternative versions of self-identity stories, V5.6); or to develop the range of escape or avoidance behaviours above (ACT, 'experiential avoidance'). Many hobbies and sources of entertainment or excitement fill this void.

The range of behaviours therefore include many mentioned earlier (see Chapter 3), including mixtures of the three alternatives above (distraction, reframing discourses, and alternative activities). These either seem to help reduce the suffering or even if they do not, they provide opportunities for new discourses (especially self-identity stories) that might help in time.

Such activities include joining in social groups to change a person's world in some new way, entertainments of all sorts, music, concerts, travel, crafts, performance, arts, study, reading, alterative religions, and general activities like walking, sports, or yoga. These might not rescue people from really bad life situations, but they can help through a myriad of ways for the people I am trying to describe in this category, those who feel they have to 'put up with it'. They might never know the hidden societal origins of their life dissatisfactions.

I briefly outlined in Chapter 5 many possible outcomes of such activities that could be 'therapeutic'. I also discussed how the effects might not be about the activity itself nor the naming given to the activity. Whatever it was that got you to try this activity might be the change to your bad situation that helps. That is, some change has already led the person to carry this out *at all*, and how that was done might be the strongest force in itself for bigger change (Guerin, 2005)

So, in terms of changing your bad situational contexts, doing any of the activities just mentioned could help because they do the following:

- Move your behaviour away from language-based conflicts.
- Get you out of the bad situations for a while.
- Unblock alternatives you could not do in the bad situation.
- Unlock alternative discourses and thoughts.
- Give new alternatives for behaviour and thinking.
- Provide possible new social relationships or break out of the old ones.
- Provide escape by getting out of the physical settings and what they shape.
- Provide escape from the monitoring and evaluation by others.
- Provide opportunities for new situations to be in.
- Provide opportunities for secrecy when back in the bad situation.
- Allow opportunities for change—some change has already led the person to carry this out *at all*, and how that was done might be the strongest force in itself (Guerin, 2005).
- Provide new life possibilities through meeting new people (resource–social relationship pathways).
- Provide new stories and other discourses for their normal audiences about this new activity.
- The person gains useful new discourses from listening to those involved in the new activity (could be advice, alternative possibilities, stories about others in similar bad situations).
- Allow for more engagement in life in a general sense.

So if someone takes up just plain walking, aside from the physical health benefits, there can be a myriad of other useful changes that might help their life, and not just the issues that are currently labelled 'mental health'.

The list above gives you some new ways of viewing how *walking* can help change people bad situations in life, up to a point. If your bad situation in life is being limited by the way patriarchy works on us all, then walking will not change that, but you might find some ways to alleviate, distract, or make smaller discourse changes for the better.

Bad life problems with hidden bad societal situations

We now get to the problem of behaviours shaped by the broad societal systems that control our lives through restricting and stratifying opportunities of all sorts. The effect of these is usually hidden from individuals, and a good 'sociological imagination' is needed (Mills, 1959). Our societies *create* many of these bad situations for people in life, which are extremely difficult to change, and indeed society could be seen to 'intentionally' make it difficult to change these bad situations.

For interventions, therefore, we need to move people into *social activism* or nothing will really change (Alinsky, 1971; Boyle, 2010; Chomsky, 2013; Doyle, 2005; Fleming, 2016; Greer, 2011; Guerin, 2010; Leonard & Sunkara, 2016; Leugi & Guerin, 2016; Macnamara, 2012; McBay, Keith, & Jensen, 2011; McCaslin, 2005; Mills, 2015; Neysmith, Bezanson, & O'Connell, 2005; Shukaitis, Graeber, & Biddle, 2007; Vestergren, Drury, & Chirac, 2019; Wilkinson & Pickett, 2010). In the meanwhile, we can only work to improve life for specific individuals and communities, or else distract them from the suffering.

In general then, to solve many of the world's bad situations we must change our society's ways of regulating and limiting our lives and our life opportunities. This means that to seriously reduce 'mental health' issues, we must all work towards better equality in our societies, stop limiting life opportunities based on when and where you were born, reduce privileges based on birth, and improve those conditions (such as our physical environments), which will in turn improve life for everyone (Kinderman, 2019; Smail, 2005; Stiglitz, 2013).

Here I will try and make small suggestions along these lines to counteract for the effects of capitalism and bureaucracy. In the next chapter we will look at the effects of colonization and patriarchy.

The life conditions produced by modernity

We cannot easily observe the nature of the pressures, stresses, and blockers arising from the conditions of Western modernity, not just because we are observing badly and non-contextually, but because they are new, generalized, and abstract to talk about. So, people who suffer most badly from these contexts are *not* poor observers, bad information processors, weak, or stupid; they are trying to live in maladaptive contexts that are not always visible and that provide no easy solutions, and for which we have no historical precedents to follow for solutions (Guerin, 2016, 2017). The way that people live in modern developed societies is relatively new, untried, global for the first time, and not yet fully tested.

They are solvable problems and conflicts, however, but they must be seen in the broader context that *our social and economic relationships in the conditions of modernity are no longer nurturing good environments for most people, people can no longer resolve their conflicts easily in the modern world, and we have no history of ways to solve these problems.*

For me the two main changes (V5.3) in life situations arise from the effects of capitalism and bureaucracy limiting what we can do (and how we might escape), and the huge changes from these in how our social relationships are now run (Guerin, 2016). Almost all our life activities, and especially those involving how we get life resources, are now based on stranger relationships rather than family relationships. This means, to give but a few examples:

- Our conflict situations are very different and hence our 'mental health' outcomes are very different.
- Avoidance and escape from relationship conflicts is very easy in modernity—having relationships with strangers makes this easier, as does the compartmentalization of our lives—but escaping does not necessarily provide alternative resources that the strangers were providing.
- We have lost the skills to engage with our social relationships since our skills are now honed on reciprocity through the exchange of money.
- We have lost the skills to engage with our physical environment since our skills are honed on what pays a salary and because we purchase the labour of others to make up for the skills we have lost.
- More of the thoughts 'popping into our heads' arise from, and involve, strangers and acquaintances.
- Conflicts or problem behaviours are difficult to resolve within stranger relationships. We tend to either give up or call the police—either is stressful.
- The issues, coping strategies, and stresses from those strangers are much more difficult to deal with because we need to work primarily in words (contractual relations), there are no clear social processes, and there is little that is concrete.
- People often have difficulty with stranger conflicts because they do not know how to persuade strangers or deal with them in contractual ways, since there is no history and the only form of reciprocity is exchanging money.
- We are far more likely to be worrying about conflicts to do with strangers, a few close friends, acquaintances, and anonymous bureaucracies than with our wider family now (of course there are exceptions).

So welcome to the twentieth and twenty-first centuries. So much of our lives, relationships, and resources are tied up with, and networked by, people we do not really know, and people who in turn do not know each other or our families, and who are not easily accountable to any of those others.

There are many good and fun relationships of course, but there are so many unknown relationships to worry about too, including strangers, dangerous random strangers, anonymous strangers in bureaucracies and in charge of organizations. This is, I suggest, the origin of both the force on our thinking, talking, and actions that is called the 'generalized other' in sociology, and the vague feelings of anxiety, doubt, and depression or hopelessness that plague us all in modernity.

We need to be clear that what we call 'mental health' in this modern era is new, and stems explicitly and directly from people's attempts to cope with the massive changes to social relationships and resource distribution (economics), and from having to do this without much guidance because we have not tried it before in history. The capitalist and bureaucratic systems also mean that so much of life we cannot understand and will never understand because it is abstracted and generalized.

Here are some examples from 'real life' of the bad events that now occur in modernity:

- You missed out on some fun and excitement because you did not have the money.
- All the best things you like to do rely on having money.
- Social relationships all feel 'meaningless' because money is used for everything and little is exchanged between friends except talk.
- You can become independent of familial, cultural, and societal patterns and can buy your way out of situations if you have capital.
- You can develop lots of new stranger relationships in most areas of life without involving any of your other social relationships.
- You feel like a self-contained individual who does not really need other people.
- You have less need to remain near to your family, and would consider moving a long way away from them if necessary.
- Life sometimes focuses more on 'self' and relations to economic networking than to family and friends.
- You can rarely do anything spontaneously and completely fun because there will be bureaucratic forms and measures needed (to protect other strangers from being sued usually).
- You could live, mostly, without human contact, so why bother with people?
- How many activities or hobbies can you do without money?
- You constantly feel like you are being cheated in monetary exchanges.
- What has happened when you have had conflicts over money with strangers involved?
- You prioritize money over people a lot of the time.
- You have spent more time learning skills to buy, shop, and sell than on learning any social skills.

- You find yourself competing with others even on trivial things, even competing with family.
- Have you been excluded from some networks of social relationships because you did not have much money?
- Do you have many anxieties over your finances, future life finances, or the monetary system not working? What if credit cards suddenly stopped working?
- You are worried that you do not have 'marketable' skills and abilities so there is anxiety over your future.
- You were told that the activities you enjoy the most and those involved in developing good social relationships will not be 'marketable' ("There is no future in doing that") so you must treat them as secondary and concentrate your life on developing 'marketable' skills.

And so, we are all trying desperately to deal with life situations that not only have had little human history from which people might have learned some good solutions, but for which there are no real answers anyway except to change the larger systems, which is unlikely to happen soon. And families cannot really help us anymore in the way they once could, since our resources come through strangers. This is the real context for mental health in modernity and our current treatments are just a tiny discursive Band-Aid in all this (Smail, 2005).

Effects of capitalism and how to help individuals and groups survive

The following list includes 25 common effects of capitalism on people (Guerin, 2016, 2017) and some simple ways we might counter them. I have mixed personal actions and social actions since we need to do both. Both Indigenous and feminist therapies have found that even joining in relevant social activism has some benefits for clients, probably from those changes listed in Chapter 5, which are concurrent with any sort of change process.

1. *Relies on a stable social system to maintain the monetary system.*
   - Disrupt the system.
   - Make some exchanges not necessarily with money.
   - Make some exchanges never with money.
   - Use alternative systems to weaken capitalism, such as sharing or bartering.
   - Find alternatives to banking.

2. *Those using money must stay within the monetary system for the money to be able to do things (have value).*
   - Avoid money by using other exchanges.
   - Make some things and events not purchasable with money at all.
   - Find alternatives to banking.
   - Exchange or barter using activities rather than 'things'.
3. *People develop good knowledge of the behaviour of money rather than the behaviour of people.*
   - Start teaching new people skills.
   - Start teaching people skills for strangers that are not competitive.
   - Start making stronger relationships with your common strangers.
   - Exchange or barter using activities rather than 'things'.
4. *Parties in monetary transactions can complain about the value given for an exchange since the dollar value is arbitrary.*
   - Ignore monetary value, pay what you think is fair or affordable.
   - Opt out of money systems of exchange.
   - Charge people what they can afford.
   - Charge people based on their opportunities in life.
5. *If conflict occurs then higher authorities can be brought in such as police and courts, thus removing the exchange from being an interpersonal exchange.*
   - Try and keep conflicts local where safe and fair.
   - Avoid using bureaucracies where safe and fair.
   - Build protocols for local conflict resolution that are just but not bureaucratic.
6. *The same item is exchanged (money).*
   - Barter.
   - Exchange other items for payments.
   - Exchange labour for payment in new ways.
   - Exchange or barter using activities rather than 'things'.
7. *Can be used to prevent any social relationship.*
   - Make exchanges more based on relationships.
   - Build stronger relationships in your exchanges with strangers (but not for discounts).
8. *Promotes individualism.*
   - If using money then try working with groups when safe (share more).
   - Share 'possessions' more.
9. *Promotes nuclear families.*
   - Support extended families.
   - Build stronger relationships with distant kin.

- Allow others into families where safe.
- Exchange or barter using activities rather than 'things'.

10. *Promotes dispersal of families.*
    - Find local employment or engagement where possible.
    - Build systems for local engagement.

11. *Facilitates indirect types of exchange.*
    - Build direct exchanges where possible.
    - Weigh up the cost of exchanges for arbitrary substitution where possible.

12. *Allows action at a distance (Weber).*
    - Promote things and events that cannot be abstracted at a distance.
    - Rediscover the local and immediate things and events in your ecology.

13. *All types of services can become valued (Weber).*
    - Demarcate things and events not available with money.
    - Find other ways to value items.

14. *Facilitates hoarding as a means of offsetting future risk (Weber). want less.*
    - Rely on groups for hoarding.
    - Rely less on bought items, self-sufficiency.
    - Exchange or barter using activities rather than 'things'.

15. *The transformation of all economic advantages into the ability to control money (Weber).*
    - Find ways to distribute resources without money.
    - Share so economic advantage not as important.

16. *Allows small groups to become independent of the larger society if they are wealthy enough (Weber).*
    - Distribute wealth more evenly.

17. *Allows individuals to become independent of groups and society, thereby facilitating forms of individualism and individual personality (Simmel).*
    - Establish group resources not available with money.
    - Reaffirm the social basis for money.

18. *Allows interactions devoid of any other social relationship (Simmel).*
    - Find new ways to engage in stranger relationships.
    - Exchange or barter using activities rather than 'things'.

19. *In this way (and points 7, 8, 9, 10, and 12 above) the use of money facilitates and encourages single-obligation contracts and interactions between strangers rather than family.*
    - Avoid single-obligation relationships.
    - New ways to encourage families and multi-exchange relationships.

20. *Promotes rational calculation, which has both good and bad effects (Simmel).*
    - Add social and moral bottom line to calculations.
21. *Is the basis for abstract thinking (Simmel).*
    - Add social and moral bottom line to calculations.
22. *Gives freedom to do what you like—if you have money (Simmel).*
    - Show limits of economic freedom.
    - Allow or arrange more activities not reliant on money.
23. *Makes most of life substitutable (Simmel).*
    - Add social and moral bottom line to calculations.
    - Be clear of substitutions done through money and abstraction.
24. *Produces a blásé attitude that makes life dull and grey (Simmel).*
    - Encourage direct engagement with people and ecology not reliant on money.
25. *Quality disappears to some extent because money is only quantity.*
    - Discern quality where applicable and do not make it cost more.
    - Encourage self-sufficiency and building of producing quality independent of money.
    - Exchange or barter using activities rather than 'things'.

Effects of bureaucracy and neoliberalism and how to help individuals and groups survive

Modernity also has a strong focus on conducting societal governance as far as possible through rational rules (language-based and anti-social, V5.1) using standardized procedures. Such bureaucracies shape a lot of depressive and anxious outcomes, even though their effects are difficult to observe (Cosgrove & Karter, 2018; Graeber, 2015; Odell, 2019; Richardson, Bishop, & Garcia-Joslin, 2018; Verdouw, 2017).

Here are some of the potential bad situations *created* by bureaucracies:

- Bureaucracies work by following written rules to control people's behaviours, but words cannot fully describe life (V4.7).
- Bureaucracies can only work if they can check that people are following rules. Bureaucracies therefore need to build strong monitoring systems therefore but these can cause more bad situations for people. Monitoring systems are then the responsibility of other bureaucracies, which only compounds all the problems.
- The bureaucratic rules in principle are perfectly transparent but most of life cannot fit exactly with any verbally based rules so negotiations and interpretations are still always needed.

- Because bureaucracies require working with strangers and not family, there is little chance to make any decisions based on contextual evidence.
- Because bureaucracies require working with strangers and not family, secrecy and lying are also easy since you do not usually have to see the bureaucrats again.
- Unknown strangers therefore control a lot of our resources and how we manage our social relationships; parts of our lives are controlled by anonymous strangers and how our lives get put into words.
- You will often not see the bureaucrats again since this is discouraged and they are rotated, so all ongoing details of your context are left to written accounts or disappear in the system.
- Once rules are written it is difficult to change or 'sway' contextual details that do not fit.
- Rules are made by those already in positions of power, usually the privileged.
- Both the bureaucrats and the government have no further obligations to people beyond the rules ("That is beyond my jurisdiction").
- Bureaucracies have the police and military systems to enforce their rules in the long run; while not used often, the threat to clients is bad.
- Because it is rule following reciprocated through money, bureaucracy can be done at a distance so no human contact is involved; especially with digital means.
- The bureaucrats themselves are personally free and subject to authority only with respect to their impersonal official obligations; out of hours they can forget their work (and you).
- The bureaucrats are organized in a clearly defined hierarchy of departments, and each department has a clearly defined sphere of competence in the legal sense; they can therefore defer or escape responsibility upwards and to other departments, as well as to the rules themselves.
- Because of all the above, most people find ways of evading or escaping part of the bureaucratic systems in place, but this in itself creates bad situations because of the monitoring and enforcement systems.

So, for those people in bad situations from which 'mental health' behaviours have arisen, we need to focus on helping them with these effects of bureaucracies even though it this not seen as part of 'normal' Western therapies (except social work). There are two problems here, in fact:

- Having our lives run through bureaucracies can cause all the bad situations above.

- Any of the other bad life situations usually require working through bureaucracies (including the mental health systems), which exacerbates the problems; many report that having to work through bureaucratic systems is as bad as the original problem.

As a broader plan, we come back to social and societal activism. If we want to help people avoid or at least cope with bad situations around bureaucracies, we need to find ways to replace or modify the huge bureaucratic systems that currently control our experiences and behaviours. Replacing the whole system of verbal rules capturing, describing, and controlling our lives (V5.1) will take longer, and alternatives are not easy with a large population. Here are some examples of smaller changes:

- From V5.1, we can try and put the *social* relationships back into the current 'rational' systems, which is not the same as making them 'irrational'; they are not mutually exclusive.
- Some solutions can *modify* the bureaucracies, for example, by giving every client an ally paid for by the system, who can develop more of a social relationship and learn about the person's context more. There are dangers in this, obviously, but no worse than the current system, I believe.
- We need to make policies and the bureaucratic implementation of those policy rules more *context sensitive*, with policies not built entirely on the 'rational' evidence base but on a base of contextual analysis— *context-driven policy* (Guerin & Guerin, 2018).
- We need implementations of policy that allow and even encourage *rules to match with individuals' contexts* rather than retain an unnecessary rigidity.

References

Alinsky, S. D. (1971). *Rules for radicals: A pragmatic primer for realistic radicals.* New York, NY: Vintage.

Boyle, M. (2010). *The moneyless man: A year of freeconomic living.* London: Oneworld Publications.

Chomsky, N. (2013). *On anarchism.* London: Penguin.

Cosgrove, L., & Karter, J. M. (2018). The poison in the cure: Neoliberalism and contemporary movements in mental health. *Theory & Psychology, 28,* 669–683.

Daniels, R. (1981). *Blues guitar: Inside & out.* Port Chester, NY: Cherry Lane Music.

Doyle, T. (2005). *Environmental movement in majority and minority worlds: A global perspective.* London: Rutgers University Press.

Fleming, D. (2016). *Lean logic: A dictionary for the future and how to survive.* Hartford, VT: Chelsea Green.

Glasper, I. (2006). *The day the country died: A history of anarcho punk 1980–1984.* London: Cherry Red Books.

Graeber, D. (2015). *The utopia of rules: On technology, stupidity, and the secret joys of bureaucracy.* London: Melville House.

Greer, J. M. (2011). *The wealth of nature: Economics as if survival mattered.* Gabriola Island, BC: New Society Publishers.

Guerin, B. (2005). *Handbook of interventions for changing people and communities.* Reno, NV: Context Press.

Guerin, B. (2010). A framework for decolonization interventions: Broadening the focus for improving the health and wellbeing of Indigenous communities. *Pimatisiwin: A Journal of Indigenous and Aboriginal Community Health, 8,* 61–83.

Guerin, B. (2016). *How to rethink human behavior: A practical guide to social contextual analysis.* London: Routledge.

Guerin, B. (2017). *How to rethink mental illness: The human contexts behind the labels.* London: Routledge.

Guerin, P., & Guerin, B. (2018). Mobility and the sustainability of remote Australian Indigenous communities: A review and a call for context-based policies. *Australian Community Psychologist, 29,* 23–37.

Kaemmer, J. E. (1989). Social power and music change among the Shona. *Ethnomusicology, 33,* 31–45.

Kinderman, P. (2019). *A manifesto for mental health: Why we need a revolution in mental health care.* London: Palgrave Macmillan.

Klein, N. (2019). *On fire: The (burning) case for a green new deal.* New York, NY: Simon & Schuster.

Leonard, S., & Sunkara, B. (2016). *The future we want: Radical ideas for a new century.* London: Metropolitan Books.

Leugi, G. B., & Guerin, B. (2016). To spark a social revolution behavior analysts must embrace community-based knowledge. *Revista Brasileira de Terapia Comportamental e Cognitiva, 18,* 73–83.

Macnamara, L. (2012). *People & permaculture: Caring and designing for ourselves, each other and the planet.* East Meon, UK: Permanent Publications.

McBay, A., Keith, L., & Jensen, D. (2011). *Deep green resistance: Strategy to save the planet.* New York, NY: Seven Stories Press.

McCaslin, W. D. (Ed.) (2005). *Justice as healing: Indigenous ways. Writings on community peacemaking and restorative justice from the Native Law Centre.* St Paul, MN: Living Justice Press.

Mills, C. (2015). The psychiatrization of poverty: Rethinking the mental health-poverty nexus. *Social and Personality Psychology Compass, 9,* 213–222.

Mills, C. W. (1959). *The sociological imagination.* Oxford: Oxford University Press.

Neysmith, S., Bezanson, K., & O'Connell, A. (2005). *Telling tales: Living the effects of public policy.* Halifax, NS: Fernwood Publishing.

Odell, J. (2019). *How to do nothing: Resisting the attention economy.* London: Melville House.

Purcell, N. J. (2003). *Death metal music: The passion and politics of a subculture.* London: MacFarland.

Richardson, F. C., Bishop, R. C., & Garcia-Joslin, J. (2018). Overcoming neo-liberalism. *Journal of Theoretical and Philosophical Psychology, 38*, 15–28.

Rowe, P. (2018). *Heavy metal youth identities: Researching the musical empower-ment of youth transitions and psychosocial wellbeing.* London: Emerald Publishing.

Rowe, P., & Guerin, B. (2018). Contextualizing the mental health of metal youth: A community for social protection, identity and musical empowerment. *Journal of Community Psychology, 46*, 1–13.

Scott-Heron, G. (2000). *Now and then.* London: Canongate.

Shukaitis, S., Graeber, D., & Biddle, E. (2007). *Constituent imagination: Militant investigations/collective theorization.* Edinburgh: AK Press.

Smail, D. (2005). *Power, interest and psychology: Elements of a social materialist understanding of distress.* London: PCCS Books.

Stiglitz, J. E. (2013). *The price of inequality.* London: Penguin.

Taylor, J. (2017). *Songs my enemy taught me.* London: Out-Spoken Press.

Truong, F. (2018). *Radicalized loyalties: Becoming Muslim in the West.* London: Polity.

Varas-Díaz, N., & Scott, N. (Eds.) (2016). *Heavy metal music and the communal experience.* New York, NY: Lexington Books.

Verdouw, J. J. (2017). The subject who thinks economically? Comparative money subjectivities in neoliberal context. *Journal of Sociology, 53*, 523–540.

Vestergren, S., Drury, J., & Chirac, E. H. (2019). How participation in collective action changes relationships, behaviours, and beliefs: An interview study of the role of inter- and intragroup processes. *Journal of Social and Political Psychology, 7*, 75–99.

Wilkinson, R., & Pickett, K. (2010). *The spirit level: Why greater equality makes societies stronger.* New York, NY: Bloomsbury Press.

8 Interventions for 'mental health' symptoms produced by colonization and patriarchal bad situations

In the approaches to psychology and mental health treatments over the last 100 years, many groups have fared badly. For most of those in some sort of 'oppressed' lifeworld, it has been clear that sorting something out in the 'mind' of the 'client' was not solving the problem, even if it brought temporary relief through distraction (Fanon, 1963). Many of these same groups could not afford the services of psychologists and psychiatrists anyway, even if they thought this might be of help.

The major groups who could more clearly see their bad situations as the source of their problems were the poor, the colonized, the slaves and descendants of former slaves, people of colour living in the white world, females, and people of non-binary sexual identity. These categories were all mixed as well. However, as mentioned in Chapter 1, governments had already appointed the medical profession (and later clinical psychology) to have the power of interpreting and 'treating' any out-of-the-ordinary behaviours that other professionals could not fix. But they were usually better trained in mythology than in sociology.

Thus all of these groups were frequently locked up (often involuntarily) in institutions when they were behaving in ways that no professionals could understand, with the psychiatrists providing abstract, brain-based theories to 'explain' what was wrong, or later the psychologists using abstract theories or everyday loose terms (Pathway 1).

This chapter will briefly examine what has been written and said about two of these oppressed groups: the colonized and women. I am no expert on these groups and have even less experience and knowledge about the others mentioned above. The work remains to be done.

What I am trying to do, however, is to see what we can glean about how some went about *trying to change the societal environments and bad situations* with these groups, in order to deal with 'mental' health issues. Unlike capitalism and bureaucracy effects, it has been clear to these groups, even if not to the professionals working with them, that they were not creating these bad situations themselves in their 'minds', but that the wider society was directly responsible. This follows W. I. Thomas's famous 'misguided' quote: "If men define situations as real, they are real in their consequences" (Thomas & Thomas, 1928, p. 572; see also V5.9). The whole idea that they could just 'change their minds' and thereby get rid of their suffering was clearly wrong, but they had little power to do anything about this (Smail, 2005).

In this sense, there are debates over how to 'decolonize' psychology so that Indigenous and other 'oppressed' groups can fare better (Guerin, 2010, 2012; Waldram, 2004). My view, however, is that 'psychology' in its current form (Pathway 1) is *incompatible* with both understanding the bad situations of such people and also their discourses and practices (V1, V4). We will never decolonize psychology in its current Pathway 1 form, we need to change psychology itself first (hence V4.1 and beyond).

Indigenous approaches: colonization and its aftermath

The colonization of the world to gain resources so that a few countries could prosper, primarily European countries including Britain, Spain, Portugal, Belgium, and Germany, left a trail of havoc for those peoples living in colonized countries. In my view, colonization has not stopped but it is now being done through economic blackmail and dependency—one country gains resources from another while leaving the original residents in a poorer and dependent situation (Klare, 2012).

In general, when the first waves of *overseas colonization* occurred (all the Indigenous peoples within Europe and the Middle East had already been suppressed under the earlier 'empires'), most of the world was living in sub-sistence economies within kin-based communities, and frequently traded among themselves (Wolf, 1982). These were not completely peaceful of course, but subsistence living generally promotes stability rather than the permanent growth of both population and resources that are necessary for capitalism and heavily promoted.

What were the bad situations for Indigenous peoples created by colonization?

There is no space for a history of colonization here. In some ways, this is not as important as it might seem, but this is only because if you are working in or alongside Indigenous groups all their histories will be different, and a general history will not help much. *You must find out the local histories and the effects of colonization in those specific places.* What I will try and do is provide some general categories to begin this dialogue.

, main effects on Indigenous peoples arising from coloniza-
ιe following:

- _ *ies*:
  - Violence.
  - Genocide.
  - Murder.
  - Disease.
  - Neglect.
  - Incarceration for not accepting the changes imposed.
  - Forced into new social groups.
  - Removal of children and incarceration of adults.
- *Economic*:
  - Removed subsistence living and hence produced dependencies.
  - Imposed a capitalist economic system for producing and distributing resources.
  - Country taken away and usually made unproductive for subsistence living.
  - Resource production dependent upon colonizers.
  - Resource distribution dependent upon colonizers and restricted, usually made contingent on obedience.
  - Direct access to resources required adopting new practices.
  - All the properties of capitalism are imposed (V5.3).
- *Community*:
  - Community organization and functions dismantled.
  - Cultural practices actively prevented or dismissed.
  - Imposition of Western/Christian cultural practices.
  - Massive discrimination and racism effects by settler populations, leading to exclusion from social relationships and hence from resources.
  - Paternalism produced by imposed dependencies.
- *Social relationships*:
  - Families broken and children taken.
  - Subsistence provision dismantled, which held families together in life pathways.
  - Imposed multiple stranger relationships to access resources.
- *Language use*:
  - Indigenous languages prohibited or minimized.
  - Indigenous languages unable to get resources anymore.
  - Imposed new languages to get things done.
  - Beliefs used within Indigenous groups reframed in new and disparaging ways.

- *Control of resources and social relationships*:
    - Many strategies imposed to control Indigenous resource access, together with directly controlling social relationships.
    - All effects were really for this end, directly or indirectly.
    - Resource distribution and social relationships funnelled through imposed bureaucratic and other administration controls.
    - Forced into new societal patterns and rules (Western patriarchy, rules, practices).
    - Total control of land, resources, and social relationships forced under the control of a Western government system, with no Indigenous exceptions allowed.
- *Control of 'minds'*:
    - In the current approach these are included within language and cultural controls imposed, but they are worth singling out separately. As both our talking and our thinking arise from the discourses around us, Indigenous peoples' talk and thinking gradually became 'full of' other languages and practices. This is especially so when Indigenous languages were prohibited or allowed to weaken. So, all of the above effects of colonization also led to talking and thinking in the Western ways that become imposed—both the languages themselves and the categories, ideas, assumptions, beliefs, etc.
    - Indigenous peoples are therefore correct to emphasize a colonization of the mind (Thiong'o, 1986) since it is shaped through difficult-to-see societal discourses and forced usage of grammars and beliefs. One of the major colonialization effects was that Western education became necessary for obtaining resources, because a knowledge of Western skills and science were prioritized. Since education was forced into the colonizers' languages this became a hugely difficult pathway for Indigenous peoples everywhere. Many children were forced into this education 'for their own benefit', which made 'sense' from the colonizers' view since all advances in resource production and distribution now required a Western education.

Sadly, the situation now is pretty much the same as above:

- The overt *brutalities* are mostly kept in check, except for police brutalities that still occur, but with *neglect* as a the most common remaining brutality.
- *Economically* the world is currently dominated by capitalism and its effects, so Indigenous access to resources requires participation; this

includes forming and maintaining the stranger relationships necessary, since without these resources are very limited.

- *Communities* never fully recovered from colonization, so they are still in various stages of disrepair (but I like to think still fixable). Colonization of communities also meant that monitoring and control of children and adults weakened so a number of other bad situations were made more possible. Without the subsistence economy and intense sharing, the communities weakened, and now with access to money children are more independent of the community.

- *Social relationships* changed in similar ways to the above with family members joined in some language and cultural practices but without the strong resource base of subsistence and sharing. Sharing is common but gets confusing with the dominant use of money to get things done. So while many Indigenous communities and families would like to be in stronger relationships, this is made difficult because of the other colonization effects and limits on resource production and distribution within families and communities.

- *Language use* has in some cases improved through revitalizing Indigenous languages, but languages only 'work' through getting people to do things and reciprocation. With all the limits imposed on resource production and distribution by the capitalist economy this makes it difficult to keep languages active since most reciprocity now occurs through money. The questions now need to be asked: What are we going to do together with this Indigenous language of ours? How can we help each other with this Indigenous language of ours rather than through the colonizers' language and economic system?

- *Control of resources and social relationships* is still very much in the hands of the colonizers. Through removing the Indigenous resource bases by claiming the land and imposing economic systems, Indigenous peoples are still reliant on the colonizers' practices to get resources, as individuals rather than as communities. Control of social relationships by the colonizers has mostly stopped as a direct strategy, but indirectly through discrimination and stratification of opportunities it remains strongly in place.

- *Control of 'minds'* continues with the colonizers' language made compulsory in education and as the dominant language in government and bureaucratic rules. This still means that the 'thinking' of Indigenous peoples arises from those dominant colonizers' languages and all the abounding discourses. Even treating the behaviours that arise from all of these bad situations is done within a Western system of language, DSM categories, and talking therapies.

What behaviours arise from these bad colonization situations and how might we change them?

Most of the DSM behaviours occur but not because there are similar brain or cognitive issues. Rather, as explained in Chapter 3, when trying to survive in bad situations in which most of the possible alternative behaviours are blocked, people will seize upon whatever is available and these behaviours will therefore be similar in many bad situations. All the other behaviours found from trying to survive bad situations will also have been shaped.

When you read all the effects of colonization, and add in the effects of the imposed capitalism and bureaucracy that went hand in hand with colonization, all the ways of changing this are really already spelt out in Indigenous agendas worldwide:

- *Self-determination*: control of social relationships and language use.
- *Return of land and country*: control of resource bases and therefore the basis of social relationships.
- *Community development and social action*: instead of fixing the brain or mind (Guerin & Guerin, 2012).

It is naïve to think that Indigenous peoples can be happy and content 'in themselves' while still living in appalling and oppressed conditions. As we saw in the last chapter, things will not be better for 'mental health' until the societal systems have been changed, since they are causing the bad situations and also blocking behaviours and strategies that could help Indigenous peoples to escape them. In the words of Martin Luther King:

> Any religion that professes to be concerned about the souls of men and is not concerned about the slums that damn them, the economic conditions that strangle them and the social conditions that cripple them is a spiritually moribund religion awaiting burial.
>
> (King, 1987, p. 66)

The same applies to therapies and other 'mental health' interventions, if they do not try and fix the person's bad life situations then it is all just fictional interior decoration.

Indigenous interventions

As always happens, Indigenous interventions for stress and conflict depend on resources and the social relationships. Because the social groups in

Indigenous communities are run through cooperating families, the problems and issues are dealt with by families. This happens in very many different ways, because there are very many different resources and social relationship contexts for these groups.

There have been many attempts to find 'Indigenous' treatments. Most essentialize and put the 'cause' on either 'being Indigenous' itself, or on some 'inner abilities' (partly summarized in Guerin, 2017; Guerin & Guerin, 2012). There are more and more better treatments occurring now that are developed by Indigenous peoples (for more information see: Alfred, 1999; Atkinson, 2002; Bantjes, Swartz, & Cembi, 2018; Brave Heart, 1988, 2003; Bristow, 2003; Coronado, 2005; Deloria, 1999; Dudgeon, Garvey, & Pickett, 2000; Dudgeon & Kelly, 2014; Durie, 1997, 1999; Estrada-Villalta & Adams, 2018; Fenton, 2000; Hartmann, Wendt, Burrage, Pomerville, & Gone, 2019; Hobart, 2003; Johnsdotter, Ingvarsdotter, Östman, & Carlbom, 2011; Kopua, Kopua, & Bracken, 2019; Laffey, 2003; Lapsley, Nikora, & Black, 2002; McCaslin, 2005; Mead, 2003; Nebelkopf & Phillips, 2004; Ngaanyatjarra Pitjantjatjara Yankunytjatjra Women's Council Aboriginal Corporation, 2003; Niania, Bush, & Epston, 2017; Ohnuki-Tierney, 1981; Panzironi, 2013; Phillips, 2003; Purdie, Dudgeon, & Walker, 2010; Roseman, 1991; Taitimu, Read, & McIntosh, 2018; Trout, McEachern, Mullany, White, & Wexler, 2018; Trzepacz, Guerin, & Thomas, 2014; Waitoki, Nikora, Harris, & Levy, 2014; Weaver & Brave Heart, 1999; Westerman, 2004; Wilson, 2008; Wilson & Yellow Bord, 2005; Zacharias, 2006)

I will give just two brief examples, especially since each group will be different. First, for some 'mental health' issues, *decolonization workshops* are given in New Zealand and elsewhere (Moeke-Pickering, 1998, 2010). This fully recognizes what is being said here: that *the source of the bad situations is not within the person but in society and that is what needs fixing*. Therefore, to change this you need to change society or at least try and work towards that. When people do decolonization workshops, they begin to see how colonization itself is the source of the bad situations, and not something about themselves.

As a second example, a Māori boy being treated for 'schizophrenia' and hearing voices was frightened and in a bad way (Niania et al., 2017). A Māori elder worked with the consulting psychiatrist in a successful collaboration to show the boy how he was hearing the voices of his ancestors, and that they probably had important messages he should listen to.

Feminist approaches: fixing the bad societal situations of women

In a similar way, female therapists working with women have long recognized that the 'mental health' issues were not arising from some dysfunction 'inside' woman, but from the bad life situations produced by societal patriarchies (Bennet, 2016; Brody, 1984; Brown, 1994; Chaplin, 1988; Enns, 1993; Hill, 1998; Hill & Rothblum, 1998; MacKinnon, 1989; Rosewater & Walker, 1985; Strömquist, 2014).

Treatments varied but included assisting women to be more assertive in their dealings with men, although this can backfire since patriarchy still gives men the majority of positions of power and privilege in government and the authorities. Treatments also included, in a similar way to decolonization workshops for Indigenous peoples, encouragement to actively take part in and learn from women's rights movements and more radical versions. The same idea applies here, that the bad situations are arising from modernity and the current forms of stranger patriarchy in Western societies, so women need to find ways of escaping these effects.

I will give one brief example from a reanalysis I made of a case study by Carl Jung (Guerin, 2019; Jung, 1917). There are just two points I want to make here.

First, in reading the case study it seemed clear to me that the woman involved had had her life stifled by the patriarchy of her time (about 1915), and all the activities she would have liked to have done were just not possible for a woman (e.g. to become a professional painter and have an independent job, not get married, not have children, not live with her parents). She was, however, unable to see the societal source of this with a 'sociological imagination' (Mills, 1959), but, just as importantly, neither could Carl Jung. They both had satisfactorily 'solved' her everyday problems (see Chapter 5) but she was still unhappy and depressed with life without knowing why, and still having conflicts with her female companion although neither could quite say why they were fighting.

When I analysed what was written, everything the client said about what she wanted to avoid in her life and what she still wanted to do with her life in the future, was rendered impossible only because of a nameless and anonymous (stranger-based) patriarchy. She wanted, for example, to be not married and to work as an artist, but both these goals were in effect prohibited. She did not want to live with her parents any longer and neither did she want to get married because that entailed having children and foregoing everything else she wanted to do with her life in order to raise a family and be a housewife. She could not live alone because that was not approved of either, so she and another like-minded woman lived together but had conflicts (I suggest that this conflict arose because theirs was a union of convenience and neither was really satisfied even though the alternatives were worse; Jung assumed they had 'homosexual tendencies').

Jung also did not have a sociological imagination, and indeed very little of a patriarchal imagination! When they were both puzzled as to why her unhappiness and conflicts remained, Jung resorted to 'explaining' this by a new, unobservable and extremely abstract theory of archetypes, rather than analysing the client's environments (Pathway 1).

The second interesting point from this is that from the turn of that century (early 1900s) onwards until today, the patriarchy, I believe, has changed. When therapies started (see Chapter 1), patriarchy was learned and enforced through the father of the family, and they gained a lot of power and privilege from others in society (both men and women) to do this. So, when problems occurred with enforcing rules on women, primarily wives and daughters, there was a concrete person who was responsible—the father. Society turned a blind eye to the methods of enforcing the patriarchy, and there are hints that Freud did the same since a lot of his clients' fathers were his friends. If Jung's client had lived around that earlier time the therapy would have focused on fixing the rift between father and daughter, by persuading the daughter to submit to her father most likely, using help from priests and others.

When we get to Jung's time, and this client in particular, we can see a shift towards the current stranger-based forms of patriarchy. Jung mentions nothing of his client's father being a problem, but when you look at her issues, it is society as a whole that is preventing her doing what she would like, not her father. We can imagine a fatherly voice:

> Well daughter, if it were up to me there would not be a problem, you could be a professional painter. But you need to be careful about what people *in general* think or you will get a very bad reputation *in town*!

In this way, this client shows features of *the patriarchy of our current times*, which is enacted by 'generalized others', societal norms, media, nameless bureaucrats making rules, etc. Her father did not seem to have any problems with her ideas, but she was still limited and now there was no concrete person to lay blame and rebel against—the start of a modern form of patriarchy where we do not even know who is doing it!

Jung produced another theory that I suggest is half-right. He remarks that through life we gradually become conscious or aware of what is controlling our lives and how to solve conflicts. In the 'first half' of life, he wrote, such 'individuation' revolves around local issues (see Chapter 5). I believe that he correctly also wrote that for some people (especially the artistic or wealthy) when the main life issues have been resolved (family, raising children, work, income) then people begin to think about other issues of their life beyond the local (although many just put up with it). For Jung, this was about becoming more aware of spiritual or religious issues in life, whereas I suggest that people should be developing their 'sociological imagination' and becoming aware of the societal and historical contexts that have shaped their life. For me, the 'individuation' Jung promoted was a fictional or otherwise abstract substitute, but perhaps helpful as a distraction. Rather, I argue that it would be better to begin to become aware of all the social, economic, cultural, societal, and patriarchal contexts that shape us into what we are and what we might become.

References

I have included here those authors I have learned from to compile the material in this chapter (whether I agreed with them or not), but not explicitly cited herein.

Alfred, T. (1999). *Peace, power, righteousness: An Indigenous manifesto*. New York, NY: Oxford.

Atkinson, J. (2002). *Trauma trails, recreating song lines: The transgenerational effects of trauma in Indigenous Australia*. Melbourne: Spinifex Press.

Bantjes, J., Swartz, L., & Cembi, S. (2018). "Our lifestyle is a mix-match": Traditional healers talk about suicide and suicide prevention in South Africa. *Transcultural Psychiatry, 55*, 73–93.

Bennet, J. (2016). *Feminist fight club: A survival manual for a sexist workplace*. New York, NY: HarperCollins.

Brave Heart, M. Y. H. (1988). The return to the sacred path: Healing the historical grief response among the Lakota through a psychoeducational group intervention. *Smith College Studies in Social Work, 68*, 287–305.

Brave Heart, M. Y. H. (2003). The historical trauma response among natives and its relationship with substance abuse: A Lakota illustration. *Journal of Psychoactive Drugs, 35*, 7–13.

Bristow, F. (Ed.) (2003). *Utz' Wach'il: Health and well-being among Indigenous peoples*. London: Health Unlimited.

Brody, C. M. (1984). *Women therapists working with women: New theory and process of feminist therapy*. New York, NY: Springer.

Brown, L. S. (1994). *Subversive dialogues: Theory in feminist therapy*. New York, NY: Basic Books.

Chaplin, J. (1988). *Feminist counselling in action*. London: Sage.

Coronado, G. (2005). Competing health models in Mexico: An ideological dialogue between Indian and hegemonic views. *Anthropology & Medicine, 12*, 165–177.

Deloria, V. (1999). *Spirit & reason: The Vine Deloria Jr reader*. Golden, CO: Fulcrum Publishing.

Dudgeon, P., Garvey, D., & Pickett, H. (2000). *Working with Indigenous Australians: A handbook for psychologists*. Perth: Gunada Press.

Dudgeon, P., & Kelly, K. (2014). Contextual factors for research on psychological therapies for Aboriginal Australians. *Australian Psychologist, 49*, 8–132.

Durie, M. (1997). *Puahou: A five-point plan for improving Māori mental health*. Wellington, NZ: Māori Mental Health Summit.

Durie, M. (1999). Mental health and Māori development. *Australian and New Zealand Journal of Psychiatry*, 33, 5–12.

Enns, C. Z. (1993). Twenty years of feminist counselling: From naming biases to implementing multifaceted practice. *Counselling Psychologist*, *21*, 3–87.

Estrada-Villalta, S., & Adams, G. (2018). Decolonizing development: A decolonial approach to the psychology of economic inequality. *Translational Issues in Psychological Science*, *4*, 198–209.

Fanon, F. (1963). *The wretched of the earth*. Ringwood, VT: Penguin Books.

Fenton, L. (2000). *Four Māori korero about their experience of mental illness*. Wellington, NZ: Mental Health Commission.

Ferdinand, A., Paradies, Y., & Kelaher, M. (2012). *Mental health impacts of racial discrimination in Victorian Aboriginal communities: The Localities Embracing and Accepting Diversity (LEAD) Experiences of Racism Survey*. Melbourne: Lowitja Institute.

Fromene, R., & Guerin, B. (2014). Talking to Australian Indigenous clients with borderline personality disorder labels: Finding the context behind the diagnosis. *Psychological Record*, *64*, 569–579.

Fromene, R., Guerin, B., & Krieg, A. (2014). Australian Indigenous clients with a borderline personality disorder diagnosis: A contextual review of the literature. *Psychological Record*, *64*, 559–567.

Ganesharajah, C., & Australian Institute of Aboriginal and Torres Strait Islander Studies. (2009). *Indigenous health and wellbeing: The importance of country*. Acton, ACT: Native Title Research Unit, Australian Institute for Aboriginal and Torres Strait Islander Studies.

Grieves, V. (2009). *Aboriginal spirituality: Aboriginal philosophy, the basis of Aboriginal social and emotional wellbeing. Discussion Paper No. 9*. Darwin: Cooperative Research Centre for Aboriginal Health.

Guerin, B. (2010). A framework for decolonization interventions: Broadening the focus for improving the health and wellbeing of Indigenous communities. *Pimatisiwin: A Journal of Indigenous and Aboriginal Community Health*, *8*, 61–83.

Guerin, B. (2012). Making psychology more relevant to Indigenous students (and others): Moving causes to context and expanding social relationships to the real world. In S. McCarthy, K. L. Dickson, J. Cranney, A. Trapp, & V. Karandashev (Eds.), *Teaching psychology around the world* (vol. 3, pp. 105–115). Newcastle upon Tyne, UK: Cambridge Scholars Publishing.

Guerin, B. (2017). *How to rethink mental illness: The human contexts behind the labels*. London: Routledge.

Guerin, B. (2019). What do therapists and clients talk about when they cannot explain behaviours? How Carl Jung avoided analysing a client's environments by inventing theories. *Revista Perspectivas em Análise Comportamento*, *10*, 76–97.

Guerin, B., & Guerin, P. (2008). Relationships in remote communities: Implications for living in remote Australia. *Australian Community Psychologist*, *20*, 74–86.

Guerin, B., & Guerin, P. (2010). Sustainability of remote communities: Population size and youth dynamics. *Journal of Economic and Social Policy*, *13*, 49–79.

Guerin, B., & Guerin, P. (2012). Re-thinking mental health for Indigenous Australian communities: Communities as context for mental health. *Community Development Journal, 47*(4), 555–570.

Guerin, B., & Guerin, P. (2014). 'Mental illness' symptoms as extensions of strategic social behaviour: The case of multicultural mental health. *Rivista di Psicologia Clinica, 1*, 67–81.

Guerin, P., & Guerin, B. (2009). Social effects of fly-in-fly-out and drive-in-drive-out services for remote Indigenous communities. *Australian Community Psychologist, 20*, 8–23.

Guerin, P., Guerin, B., & Tedmanson, D. (2011). *Bureaucratic stress syndrome and remote Aboriginal communities.* Paper presented at the International Society of Critical Health Psychology 7th Biennial Conference, Adelaide, South Australia.

Guerin, P., Guerin, B., Tedmanson, D., & Clark, Y. (2009). How do we think about Indigenous mental health in rural and remote communities? *STATEing Women's Health*, 8–13.

Guerin, P., Guerin, B., Tedmanson, D., & Clark, Y. (2011). How can country, spirituality, music and arts contribute to Indigenous mental health and well-being? *Australasian Psychiatry, 19*, 38–41.

Hartmann, W. E., Wendt, D. C., Burrage, R. L., Pomerville, A., & Gone, J. P. (2019). American Indian historical trauma: Anticolonial prescriptions for healing, resilience, and survivance. *American Psychologist, 74*, 6–19.

Hill, M. (Ed.) (1998). *Feminist therapy as a political act.* New York, NY: Haworth Press.

Hill, M., & Rothblum, E. D. (Eds.) (1998). *Learning from our mistakes: Difficulties and failure in feminist therapy.* New York, NY: Haworth Press.

Hobart, A. (2003). *Healing performances of Bali: Between darkness and light.* New York, NY: Berghahn Books.

Johnsdotter, S., Ingvarsdotter, K., Östman, M., & Carlbom, A. (2011). Koran reading and negotiation with jinn: Strategies to deal with mental ill health among Swedish Somalis. *Mental Health, Religion & Culture, 14*, 741–755.

Jung, C. G. (1917). *On the psychology of the unconscious.* New York, NY: Bollington Foundation.

King, M. L. (1987). The words of Martin Luther King, Jr. New York, NY: Newmarket Press.

Kingsley, J., Townsend, M., Philips, R., & Aldous, D. (2009). If the land is healthy it makes the people healthy: The relationship between caring for country and health for the yorta yorta nation, boonwurrunga and bangerang tribes. *Health and Place, 15*, 291–299.

Klare, M. T. (2012). *The race for what's left: The global scramble for the world's last resources.* New York, NY: Picador.

Kopua, D. M., Kopua, M. A., & Bracken, P. J. (2019). Mahi a Atua: A Maori approach to mental health. *Transcultural Psychiatry, 51*(6), 850–874.

Laffey, P. (2003). Psychiatric therapy in Georgian Britain. *Psychological Medicine, 33*, 1285–1297.

Lapsley, H., Nikora, L. W., & Black, R. (2002). *'Kia Mauri Tau!' Narratives of recovery from disabling mental health problems.* Wellington, NZ: Mental Health Commission.

MacKinnon, C. A. (1989). *Toward a feminist theory of the state.* London: Harvard University Press.

McCaslin, W. D. (Ed.) (2005). *Justice as healing: Indigenous ways.* St Paul, MN: Living Justice Press.

Mead, H. M. (2003). *Tikanga Māori: Living by Māori values.* Wellington, NZ: Huia Publishers.

Mills, C. W. (1959). *The sociological imagination.* Oxford: Oxford University Press.

Moeke-Pickering, T. (1998). *Evaluation of the effectiveness of a decolonization/ anti-oppression and liberation workshop as an intervention strategy.* Hamilton, NZ: University of Waikato.

Moeke-Pickering, T. (2010). *Decolonisation as a social change framework and its impact on the development of Indigenous-based curricula for helping professionals in mainstream tertiary education organisations.* Hamilton, NZ: University of Waikato. Retrieved from http://researchcommons.waikato.ac.nz/ bitstream/10289/4148/3/thesis.pdf.

Nebelkopf, E., & Phillips, M. (Eds.). (2004). *Healing and mental health for Native Americans: Speaking in red.* New York, NY: Altamira Press.

Ngaanyatjarra Pitjantjatjara Yankunytjatjra Women's Council Aboriginal Corporation. (2003). *Ngangkari work—Anangu way: Traditional healers of Central Australia.* Black Point, NS: Fernwood Publishing.

Niania, W., Bush, A., & Epston, D. (2017). *Collaborative and Indigenous mental health therapy: Tātaihono—Stories of Māori healing and psychiatry.* London: Routledge.

Ohnuki-Tierney, E. (1981). *Illness and healing among the Sakhalin Ainu.: A symbolic interpretation.* London: Cambridge University Press.

Panzironi, F. (2013). *Hand-in-hand: Report on Aboriginal traditional medicine.* Fregon, South Australia: Anangu Ngangkari Tjutaku Aboriginal Corporation. Retrieved from www.antac.org.au.

Phillips, G. (2003). *Addictions and healing in Aboriginal country.* Canberra: Aboriginal Studies Press.

Purdie, N., Dudgeon, P., & Walker, R. (2010). *Working together: Aboriginal and Torres Strait Islander mental health and wellbeing principles and practice.* Canberra: Australian Government Printers.

Roseman, M. (1991). *Healing sounds from the Malaysian rainforest: Temiar music and medicine.* London: University of California Press.

Rosewater, L. B., & Walker, L. E. A. (Eds.) (1985). *Handbook of feminist therapy: Women's issues in psychotherapy.* New York, NY: Springer.

Smail, D. (2005). *Power, interest and psychology: Elements of a social materialist understanding of distress.* London: PCCS Books.

Strömquist, L. (2014). *Fruit of knowledge: The vulva vs. the patriarchy.* London: Virago.

Taitimu, M., Read, J., & McIntosh, T. (2018). Ngā Whakāwhitinga (standing at the crossroads): How Māori understand what Western psychiatry calls 'schizophrenia'. *Transcultural Psychiatry, 55*, 153–177.

Thiong'o, N. (1986). *Decolonising the mind: The politics of language in African literature*. London: J. Currey.

Thomas, W. I., & Thomas, D. S. (1928). *The child in America: Behavior problems and programs*. New York, NY: Knopf.

Trout, L., McEachern, D., Mullany, A., White, L., & Wexler, L. (2018). Decoloniality as a framework for Indigenous youth suicide prevention pedagogy: Promoting community conversations about research to end suicide. *American Journal of Community Psychology, 62*, 396–405.

Trzepacz, D., Guerin, B., & Thomas, J. (2014). Indigenous country as a context for mental and physical health: Yarning with the Nukunu community. *Australian Community Psychologist, 26*, 38–53.

Waitoki, W., Nikora, L. M., Harris, P., & Levy, M. (2014). *Māori experiences of bipolar disorder: Pathways to recovery*. Auckland, NZ: Te Pou o te Whakaaro Nui.

Waldram, J. B. (2004). *Revenge of the Windigo: The construction of the mind and mental health of North American Aboriginal peoples*. Toronto: University of Toronto Press.

Weaver, H. N., & Brave Heart, M. Y. H. (1999). Examining two facets of American Indian identity: Exposure to other cultures and the influence of historical trauma. *Journal of Human Behavior in the Social Environment, 2*, 19–33.

Westerman, T. (2004). Engagement of indigenous clients in mental health services: What role do cultural differences play? *Australian e-Journal for the Advancement of Mental Health, 3*, 1–7.

Wilson, S. (2008). *Research is ceremony: Indigenous research methods*. Black Point, NS: Fernwood Publishing.

Wilson, W. A., & Yellow Bird, M. (2005). *For Indigenous eyes only: A decolonization handbook*. Santa Fe, NM: School of American Research Press.

Wolf, E. R. (1982). *Europe and the people without history*. Berkeley, CA: University of California Press.

Zacharias, S. (2006). Mexican *Curanderismo* as ethnopsychotherapy: A qualitative study on treatment practices, effectiveness, and mechanisms of change. *International Journal of Disability, Development and Education, 53*, 381–400.

Index

Note: Page numbers in bold refer to **tables** and in *italics* to figures.